When Feelings Speak, LISTEN!

How To Manage Emotional Stress Using Your Emotions

07/04/2014

To James Kemp,

Best wishes for your emotional peace.

Freeda L. Moore

Freeda L. Biggs Moore, RN, MS, APN

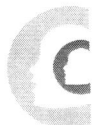

Logo designed by Eileen Glazer, Commercial Artist, Houston, Texas for Personal Counseling and Guidance Center, 1979

ISBN: 978-1-4834-0170-6 (sc)
ISBN: 978-1-4834-0169-0 (e)

Lulu Publishing Services rev. date: 6/21/2013

TABLE OF CONTENTS

ACKNOWLEDGEMENTS

First, I want to give thanks and praise to Almighty God for guiding my thoughts and abilities into organizing and writing the contents of this insightful exciting tour in an orderly, easily-flowing and understandable manner.

Sincere appreciation is extended to the many participants who shared their experiences and introspections during my mental health practice. It was a pleasure watching you grow and assisting in your development. The practice included presenting personal development workshops and private counseling to a wide range of individuals and groups, on a mission to spread the word about regaining and maintaining a status of good mental health.

Thanks also to my family: my parents, Walter and Arnesia Biggs, plus my siblings Billy, Bobby, James, Michael, Quintin and particularly Jacqueline—my only sister and best friend who was a popular Speech Pathologist in Houston. They got to hear about it all—the pluses and minuses, ups and angles, etc. It was Quintin, my youngest brother, who inspired me last summer to retrieve this manuscript from the shelf in my storage house and rewrite it. The copy of a previous version I had given to him several years ago was lost during Hurricane Ike and he was asking for another copy. Pleasantly surprised by this reminder, I did as requested and you see here the results.

A special thanks to my rock, my love, my husband, Yondell E. Moore, Sr. Throughout our years of marriage, on occasions I would mention to him about the book I had written, but he never saw it. When he finally actually saw it last summer, he just looked at me in surprise and smiled. His encouragement began then and has never dwindled. The enthusiasm, devotion of time and energy to proof-read—primarily grammatically, ask questions to assist me in clarifying, etc—all to enable me to attain this goal.

I sincerely hope you enjoy this presentation as much as I enjoyed preparing it. Be assured, there will be nuggets you can use in your quest to effectively manage your emotions, reduce emotional stress and return to a peaceful emotional status.

Thank you.

Freeda L. Biggs Moore

INTRODUCTION

Mankind has come a long way since the Stone Age in our observable styles and manners of daily living. Externally, we have advanced through scientific knowledge explosions, medical breakthroughs, a whirlwind of evolutionary technology and much, much more. Overall, we live a significant number of years longer, earn more money per person and own more material things than ever before in our history.

Yet, despite observable achievements and positive improvements in external living, all is not well among the general population. Emotional stress—an internal living issue—retains its long-standing status as the leading destroyer of human life in modern times and it is on the increase. Everyday more and more people are displaying symptoms of its disquieting effects, including:

> physical illnesses and disorders;
> mental or thinking disruptions;
> spiritual estrangements; and
> emotional disturbances.

"Progress" is the term used to describe the on-going knowledge growth, a process generating alternatives for improving and expanding current external achievements and results in changes in our everyday living styles. We can reasonably assume progress will continue for an indefinite time—uprooting the old and familiar and merging them or discarding them for the new and unfamiliar.

However, general observations and documented statistics report the number of present-day victims of emotional stress as soaring past epidemic proportions, seemingly unabated. It appears that, although we have progressed externally in how we live,

emotionally we are stifled.

What is emotional stress and how can we remedy this internal disorder? Is genuine relief possible? If so, what does it require from people to prevent it or effectively correct it?

Realistically, emotional stress concerns human feelings or emotions. Simply stated, it is internal pressure we experience resulting from build-ups in ineffectively resolved emotions.

Feelings live and function internally in organs and spaces throughout our physical body. Therefore, their conduct and activities are a very personal matter. They are components of the inherent criteria differentiating us as human beings, rather than

plant beings ... insect beings ... bird beings ...

rock beings ... fish beings ... .

Consequently, emotions enjoy a permanent position among our human characteristics. They cannot be totally eliminated from our essence. Neither can they be "dismissed" or fired from their natural duties to participate in and to influence each of our experiences throughout day-to-day living.

It is well documented throughout the literature that our human attitude consists primarily of three components: thoughts, feelings and behaviors. Extensive research continues to be performed and publicized regarding in-depth insights into the significance, mechanisms and contributions of our thoughts and thinking processes, as well as our behaviors.

However, seldom are feelings given the same platform of exposure. Most often, emotions are pushed aside or reduced to having been caused by or resulting from their two attitudinal colleagues.

Our primary objective is to present emotions from their natural status of importance in their own right that is not solely dependent upon our thoughts or behaviors—just as our Creator intended. They are separate and, at the least, equal in significance to their two partners. As such, feelings deserve and even demand separate, equal and direct attention from their owner when emotional balance or peace is our goal.

Several strategies have been recommended to conquer emotional dis-at-ease and each of these has its value. An array of information is readily accessible promoting remedies for stress using

> approaches through physical body parts (e.g., muscle-grooming exercises; jogging; dietary changes; medications; surgery; etc.);

> mental or intellectual approaches (e.g., based on the premise feelings are "caused" by our thoughts and can therefore be resolved by reviewing and adding information to our intellect—going through our thoughts. Their appeal is for us to think our way into better feelings);

> spiritual attitudes and rituals (e.g., yoga; medication; parapsychology participation;

practicing religious principles and beliefs exclusively; etc.).

While such indirect approaches to emotional stress have useful aspects, swelling statistics demonstrate that, used exclusively, their ability to sustain relief from emotional stress is short-term. They may distract us temporarily from the pains of stress, but the core of the problem— our build-ups of stressful emotions—persists. Moreover, unless effective, longer-lasting interventions are brought into our awareness—and practiced—the ineffectively resolved emotions will resume their pressuring growth into disrupting our life repeatedly at later times.

As previously stated, emotions are enjoined by our Creator to keep us attuned and informed about the internal and external worlds we live in. Their primary "duties" or "jobs" consist of two principle functions, namely to

collect information

and

deliver that information

directly to our brain for consideration as meaningful content for our decision-making process. Therefore, they will not rest until both functions are directly accomplished. In fact, their return to balance requires and even demands our underline attention.

Perhaps the time has come to approach feelings directly to successfully resolve them, rather than advancing another indirect approach. It seems reasonable a more effective and practical method of settling emotions can be achieved by "going to the horse's mouth" to straight-forwardly examine feelings on their own natural turf. Emotions have information to share from their own perspective, knowledge-base and level of astuteness, including:

- who they are (their identity);
- what is/was happening in our internal and external worlds that attracted their attention (the situation);
- when or at what point they became aroused (the information they collected from the situation, e.g., their purpose for arousal);
- once aroused, what their business with us concerns (the messages they intend to deliver to our brain for acknowledgment and consideration); plus
- how-to's for successfully settling them …

…so they can return to resting peacefully again inside us.

Within these pages, the personal management of our emotions is addressed directly. We escort you on an enlightening straightforward tour through our emotional world, traveling "behind the scenes" and on "center-stage" with emotions themselves. Along the way, we explore their basic functions; healthy and unhealthy programming; intrinsic, unique, revealing messages to us; and realistic, effective self-management strategies.

We recognize stressful feelings (e.g., anger, hurt, guilt, fear, etc.) are painful to experience. But, we firmly believe our Creator (by any of its assigned names) did not provide us with emotions merely as negative forces—to be burdens and punishments for us to endure. In our practice of psychotherapy and personal development, emotions were found to be assets to human daily living, signaling positive, supportive and quite pertinent information for us to respectfully acknowledge and attend to.

The majority of insights into emotions and their management discussed here were shared by ordinary people in a variety of self development settings. While most often participants were not acquainted with each other, certain repetitions or trends were observed in the information they shared during personal introspections. The repetitions led to the awareness people possess a common knowledge about emotions and their management that can be considered natural or inherent. Those common trends of information compose a major portion of this recording.

Some comments discussed are supported by researchers and writers throughout the literature. Others will likely sound familiar to you, though this presentation is their written debut.

<u>Please be advised that, throughout the content, words spelled using all capital letters indicate "the natural and realistic".</u>

Although emotions function without our alert awareness, ultimately they are ruled by our own voluntary control. Despite permanence in our human essence and their innate obligation to perform their "jobs", every person—intrinsically—owns the POWER necessary to manage and control the feelings we experience. POWER over our own emotions is a natural ability also included in the "package-deal" of being human.

A more detailed discussion regarding personal POWER over feelings will come later during our tour. But for now, we state with assurance by becoming aware of our feelings—with respect—and deliberately using our inherent POWER over them—we can successfully shrink aroused and stressful emotions and return them to their positions of balance inside us.

We do not pretend, to any extent, this presentation holds "all" of the answers regarding human emotions. However, we sincerely believe it significantly contributes to the body of knowledge presently known and publicly available. At best, we hope it will inspire a greater appreciation for emotions in their own right and stimulate more intensive research into feelings using more direct approaches.

PART I

WELCOME TO OUR EMOTIONAL WORLD!

For years, people have demonstrated an interest in what makes human beings "tick" and how we function. Seemingly, this information is necessary to effectively "fix" the problems we incur in our abilities to perform throughout daily living.

Those of us who concern ourselves with emotional health are particularly interested in how we conduct ourselves in our attitude, e.g., in our

> thoughts,
> feelings and
> behaviors.

Several theories have been advanced to explain these human phenomena and still more are entering the limelight today.

Thoughts, feelings and behaviors all three components form our human attitude. However, the majority of specific information circulating among the general public predominantly relates to thoughts and thinking processes, along with our observable behaviors. Emotions are seldom allowed the same visibility. Even more rarely are they discussed directly. For the most part, human emotions are overlooked as an equal partner on the attitudinal team, deserving equal time and attention.

Granted, occasionally we find inferences and indirect hints about them. Most often however, emotions are blamed on their two colleagues—our thoughts and behaviors. Hardly ever are they given full credit for existing and functioning in their own right—as uniquely separate and equally significant entities, carrying their own weight, and earning their own worth in our daily life.

Though treated to the contrary, feelings are important, powerful entities. Every phase of daily living is accompanied and influenced by our emotions. They compose the innate communications system that keeps us alert, tuned into and <u>accurately</u> informed about events occurring in our

> internal world,
> external environment and
> interpersonal involvements.

More specifically, they are the natural connecting links joining external situations and events with our internal system of awareness and responding.

Emotions really are supportive to their owner and they are our friends. Rather than continuing with limited knowledge and inadequate attention to them, we invite you on an eye-opening tour directly through our emotional world. Make yourself comfortable while we present feelings from center stage. Get better acquainted with your emotions in their own right by collecting useful insights gleaned from their own natural turf. We will share:

- reports from emotions about their purposes and how they function;
- interpretations of themselves, both positively and negatively; and
- remedies for effectively managing and returning them to balance inside us.

Before we begin, a few house rules will apply as we travel:

1) You are permitted to think for yourself.

2) You are permitted to feel and acknowledge it, particularly to yourself, but not necessarily to others.

3) You are permitted to agree or disagree with the content being presented.

4) You are permitted to "try-on" new information for size and fitness for you.

5) With the new information gleaned, you are permitted to choose among:

    a) keeping your life as is without making changes (when done with awareness, this becomes a good choice);

    b) modifying segments of your practices; or

    c) completely changing things around for yourself.

So, Welcome to Our Emotional World!

Though feelings vary in appearances and methods of expression from person to person, certain characteristics are consistent. Several general qualities are documented throughout the literature and were repeatedly revealed during personal development sessions. Because these qualities redundantly appeared, we view them as basic, fundamental FACTS about feelings.

This tour begins now with—

1. Basic FACTS About Feelings

Perhaps it would not surprise you to know,

1. <u>Without exception, every human being comes fully equipped from birth with a separate, permanent and complete set of feelings.</u>

Feelings are inherent phenomena. They are a part of the natural criteria differentiating human beings from other species of beings among the vast assortment in the universe.

Emotions exist in our essence in complete sets—exclusively. Realistically, people with missing or absent feelings simply do not exist. While human capabilities are enormous, we are limited in that we can neither create feelings nor eliminate them from our essence. Consequently, whether or not we experience each of them during our lifetime, the "seeds" of every emotion humanly possible innately reside inside each of us. Moreover, they remain permanently available for us for stimulation as indicated throughout our daily living. When not aroused, they are in "at rest" positions, still eternally available upon notice.

Each set of feelings contains some amount of every emotion in the gamut of affective responses a person can experience—ranging from the heights of ecstasy and pleasure to the depths of emotional pain (homicidal and suicidal feelings). Also, we have the natural capability to experience each emotion in its pure or raw form, as well as its various degrees or intensities.

Though feelings occupy a large portion of the emotional level of living, according to other writers their domain is shared with our natural instincts, intuitions, and hunches. Collectively, these elements contribute to the storehouse of wisdoms each of us innately possesses.

Every person exists as a complete, intact and uniquely separate human specimen in our own right, regardless of flaws and defects (more positively and correctly identified here as "areas for improvement"). Our Creator indiscriminately weaved into our essence a total package of materials rendering us eligible to be successfully classified as human, fully capable of living and functioning as whole PERSONS who are similar, yet separate from each other.

While we are social beings, our ability to qualify as human is not dependent upon anyone or anything else for affirmation. Neither are we dependent upon another person for continued life and survival. I am reminded of a popular personal development class we presented primarily for single or unmarried persons entitled "One Is A Whole

PERSON". Consequently, just as our hands, stomachs and intellects are disconnected from each other's, one person's set of feelings is detached from another person's set.

Let's look at another basic FACT about feelings.

2. Feelings are a permanent part of our daily existence.

Feelings are on-going phenomena, rather than temporarily "here today, gone tomorrow". They are alive and active in each thought we entertain, every activity we perform, and every situation we encounter, 24-hours-a-day, throughout our lifetime. Regardless of age, gender or how we conduct ourselves, our set of feelings remains incorporated into our essence for as long as we remain human.

Because they enjoy the status of permanence in our humanness, feelings cannot be removed, destroyed, gotten rid of, eliminated, etc. However, using our innate POWER over ourselves in our attitude (thoughts, feelings and behaviors), we can:

- stimulate our emotions from their resting positions inside us;
- manage the conduct of their behavior during arousal;

- control their course or direction of flow and length of time they remain aroused inside us; plus
- shrink them from overgrown postures of <u>assumed</u> control over us.

Feelings are flexible. Though they can increase in size, the good news is their owner inherently possesses the tools to alter their overgrown states and reduce them into more easily managed dimensions.

We firmly believe emotions were not incorporated into the essence of our humanness to keep us in emotional agony. On the contrary, feelings are useful, positive resources for improving the quality of daily living. They work to carry out quite healthy and responsible duties as their contribution to our overall health. Just as nerve endings in physical body parts relay information about physical comforts and discomforts, emotions transmit messages concerning our emotional,

> plus mental (thoughts and thinking processes),
> plus behavioral

states of affairs.

Feelings are naturally enjoined to

initiate,

accompany and

exert influence upon

each of our experiences throughout life, including every

thought we entertain;

feeling we experience (yes, people have feelings about feelings); and

behavior we perform.

They can function autonomously or without our alert attention and regularly demonstrate their ability to be persuasive motivators. When permitted, they have the ability to grow into appearing as though they are the controllers of our physical, mental, emotional and spiritual behaviors—the total scope of our existence.

3. Feelings transmit valuable and positive information

Feelings compose our inherent system for communicating specific messages and other relevant FACTS from our natural knowledge-pool to our brain for consideration. To be pragmatic, without a means to communicate its FACTS and insights, our innately-known information would merely be uselessly "hanging around". Emotions resolve the dilemma. Their primary, two-fold, naturally-assigned task—the central purpose for their existence—is to function in an information-collecting-and-delivering capacity.

Possibly you are aware feelings gather information. However, since delivering that information is also a primary duty, once aroused, they <u>will</u> <u>not</u> rest quietly and peacefully again for a sustained time-period until this second part of their major mission is completed. Innately, they are programmed to deliver information concerning our current experiences and intuitive knowledge people naturally hold-in-common. Furthermore, the information they offer is pertinent, reliable and beneficial to us in healthily working through daily life situations towards emotional health and calmness.

Pleasant feelings, popularly referred to as "good", inform us when we have achieved emotional balance or peace for a time. They also allow us to know, intuitively, when we are experiencing pleasure, comfort, happiness, goal achievement, safety, etc.,—when we are emotionally in harmony with person(s) and/or things in our external environment and internally with ourselves.

Feelings experienced as unpleasant or "bad" carry positive and supportive messages also. They tell us when events are occurring in our internal world (from SELF-to-SELF) and/or external involvements (SELF-to-others) that are not in our best interest.

Everyday people have demonstrated repeatedly when we allow ourselves to pause for a moment to relax, flow and listen to our feelings with open minds, among other valuable information, uncomfortable feelings have the abilities:

- to identify the offending event or person (specific-awareness);
- to describe how another person and/or external event managed to influence us emotionally—including techniques and strategies they used (other-awareness);
- to describe potential outcomes for us should we allow the aroused feeling(s) and its related problem-issues to continue, unresolved, for projected time periods into the future (SELF-prevention);

- to describe possible reactions of others if we were to practice different behaviors to resolve our problem situations (SELF-preparation);
- to provide solutions that can, in fact, lead to a return to emotional balance for us, while keeping our overall best interest uppermost in mind (SELF-protection); and
- to realistically evaluate our progress for ourselves towards effectively resolving emotional problem-issues we are living with (SELF-support).

It can be refreshing to know, assuredly, we are moving towards effectively resolving our emotional problem-issues in daily living by listening to our feelings. Let us interject here, progress is measured or demonstrated when the original unpleasant feeling is experienced as <u>less</u> and <u>less</u> intense. In addition, we can notice a reduction in the disruptive effects the stressful feeling is wielding upon our overall functions and activities. In essence, the pressure inside us exerted by the aroused emotion lightens.

4. Feelings are not subject to arbitrations and judgments.

Judgments are not applicable to feelings. Rendering verdicts to emotions, though popularly practiced, is discounting and disrespectful to ourselves and others.

Feelings are neither:

> right nor wrong;
> appropriate nor inappropriate;
> good or bad;
> proper nor improper;
> masculine nor feminine;
> childish nor mature; etc.

Emotions simply ARE. They exist for positive, supportive purposes. To repeat, they are our innate communication system, designed by our Creator, enabling us to become realistically aware and to regulate ourselves accordingly. Feelings assess and collect information to inform us about events and happenings occurring in our internal world and external involvements.

Judgments are opinions, whereas feelings are FACTS. Opinions are temporary phenomena subject to change as time proceeds and new information is integrated. They are flexible, speculative, optional and dependent upon social convention or agreement for their meaning and survival. FACTS, on the other hand, are constant, permanent phenomena. They do not rely upon our alert awareness, agreement, acceptance, nor any other human process to persist and remain true.

The information feelings carry is intended to inform and benefit the person experiencing the emotion. By allowing ourselves

> to pause for a while,
> relax and
> flow with a feeling
> without self-condemnation and restraint,

we can arrive at the facts supporting the emotion's stimulated state—the reasons or "whys" for its current prominence.

5. <u>Aroused feelings demand direct attention or recognition from their owner to be effectively resolved.</u>

To begin the healthy management of emotions, it is imperative we <u>directly</u> recognize and claim ownership of the aroused feeling to ourselves. In other words, admit to the feeling's presence and own or acknowledge it as our own property.

Directly recognizing and owning our feeling can be accomplished with a simple statement such as "I am feeling _____", completing the statement with the feeling's specific name. Vague and indefinite expressions, such as "I just don't feel 'good'" and "I don't feel 'right'" can be beginning points of sorting to identify and label the feeling.

But, they are insufficient as substitutes for the feeling's specific name-identity.

Other questions to ask yourself when seeking the specific name-identity of your feeling are "How am I feeling?" and/or "What am I feeling?" Try-on different answers until you become aware of the feeling's identity. Now, fill-in the above blank addressing the emotion by its name. In this way, the feeling knows, intuitively, you at least "see" it—a fact that provides it with some amount of immediate relief for us to enjoy.

Feelings adamantly demand direct recognition from their owner if they are to be effectively resolved. Recognition from outsiders can assist and support us in resolving our feelings, but it cannot substitute for the direct attention required from us. Realistically, outsiders are not capable of possessing any amount of genuine POWER over emotions housed in our internal set. Consequently, despite their efforts and wishes for us, it is impossible for another person and/or external things to bring about any amount of change in the status of our feelings. Their ability to even influence our emotions requires that, ultimately, we must agree with their opinion(s).

Aroused feelings are active. powerful entities. They do not tolerate being flipped off, ignored, pushed aside and forgotten by their owner. Remember, they are programmed by our Creator to gather information, as well as to deliver messages regarding their findings to us—and they fully intend to complete both missions.

While it is painful to emotions to be denied the positive attention and respect they prefer, they cannot shun their duties. Choosing not to listen to their transmissions does not permit feelings the prerogative to tuck their heads and quietly disappear. Rather than flipping, shaking or working them off, as we have erroneously learned is possible, we flip the feelings into storage sites inside us, still unresolved and hurting. Over time, the hurts accumulate and connect, one to the other, forming groups of personal hurts (e.g., emotional soft, sore or weak spots).

As examples, we may harbor collections of hurts or sore spots related to our:

> intelligence;
> coordination;
> parenting ability;
> thinking ability;
> "maleness"/ "femaleness";
> ability to speak up for ourselves;
> ability to make decisions;
> patience;
> judgment; etc.

Repeatedly neglecting hurt feelings and swallowing them as similar and again painful situations occur in daily living, add to the stored collections. Because the hurts are unresolved, they are still in their active states, constantly churning, generating heat and steam (pressure) inside us in the process.

As the collection of hurts regarding, for example, our thinking ability grows and the storage space becomes crammed, pressure is applied to surrounding structures. Several researchers throughout the literature affirm unresolved hurtful feelings we experience may eventually become obscured from us, but they do not automatically dissipate. Instead, they continue to exert subtle pressures and can, in time, result in illnesses and malfunctions throughout our body.

Collections of hurt feelings can explode to interfere with orderly functions on either of our levels of living. As examples, they can produce

physical body symptoms:
(e.g., ulcer; colitis; chest pains; elevated blood pressure; colds; headaches; joint pains; rashes; asthma; nail-biting behavior; diarrhea; constipation; urinary problems; cancer; etc.);

mental and thinking disruptions:

(e.g., memory loss; inability to concentrate; daydreaming; mental blocks; excessive forgetting; rambling, compulsive speech; indecisiveness; impulsive comments; etc.);

emotional disturbances:

(e.g., excessive worry; extreme frustration; flare-ups of confusion; overwhelming guilt; seething despair; rancorous blaming; homicidal or suicidal depression; outwardly-explosive anger; immobilizing fear; despondency; sadness; debilitating loss of energy; episodes of insanity; etc.);

spiritual limitations:

(e.g., reduced self-esteem; low self-trust; dwindled self-confidence; decreased self-appreciation; atheism; distrust of others; etc.).

I am reminded of a businessman we affectionately refer to as "the client with the contracted elbow" who came to the office for counseling. He was the epitome of a gentleman— gentle in every observable respect: softly spoken voice, a gentle handshake; displaying a permanent, soft smile; quiet, mannerly foot steps, etc. Though he entered counseling to resolve issues related to a bossy co-worker, we moved into related anger-issues while growing up pertaining to his mother. He described his mother as domineering;

physically and verbally abusive; overly protective; always prying and searching his room; etc.

Working through his anger and emotional pains (anger = hurt), over time he began releasing accumulated hurts and the elbow loosened to release the contracture. We found out his anger/hurt for his mother had frozen his elbow into a contracture to prevent striking her. After all, the external guideline he learned was "you can't hit your mother!" Neither did I, as his counselor, advocate striking the mother as a healthy solution for him.

Fortunately, the body can restore itself to health once we make a sincere decision to do so. We can relieve stressful emotional buildups through making positive decisions and taking realistic healthy actions toward balance.

Restoration for this client continued with introducing him to a different mental health guideline for practice:

"We teach others how to treat us by how
we treat ourselves".

He was encouraged to have a straightforward, unabridged conversation with his mother expressing his hurts that we practiced in fantasy the same day while at our office.

21

In addition to his hurts, when she said certain "triggers" to him, he was to inform her of his preferences for her to say. He also was to let her know that, should she chose not to honor his preferences, how he would respond. Among other options, he would:

- say aloud with fervor, "Stop it, that hurts!"—using whatever language style he chose;
- interrupt her with positive statements about himself and/or her—even if the comments are completely out of context from the current issue;
- turn and walk away leaving the room, letting her know aloud he would no longer tolerate that behavior from her (if he feels safe to leave the room).

These options could also be practiced with the bossy co-worker.

Near the end of the practice session, we let the client know it was not mandatory to have this conversation with his mother face-to-face. Regardless of his requests of her, he could not change his mother's behavior towards him. The extent of his POWER was to change his response to her messages and methodology in the interest of his own health.

To repeat for emphasis, we teach other people how to treat us by how we treat ourselves, e.g., by what we allow them to do, say and behave around us. By not objecting to offensive behaviors, our silence condones whatever they are doing. Since they cannot read our minds. the only way they will know our preferences is when we inform them!

6. <u>Feelings are seldom, if ever, logical and rational. They cannot be resolved using "Why?" questions.</u>

It is difficult, at best, to comprehend and effectively resolve feelings using "becauses" given in response to "Why's?" 'Why's?" appeal to logic, deductive reasoning, rationalization and other forms of ordered thinking. These methods interpret reality with answers to nourish our mental level of living—our intellect and thinking processes.

In contrast, feelings exist on our emotional level, where the methods of examination differ significantly. Whenever emotions are the issue, neither <u>Robert's Rules of Order</u>, the scientific method nor any other system based on logic is relevant. Therefore, asking the question 'Why?" to search for explanations and solutions for feelings is ineffective. "Why?" demands logical, orderly responses, whereas feelings are illogical and defy order.

This does not imply, by any measure, feelings are incoherent and incapable of understanding. As stated previously, the unique information they signal is difficult to relay using methods more appropriately applicable to our intellect.

To question "Why?" is unfair and discounting to feelings—our own and someone else's. It does not address emotions nor resolve them, while it carries a high probability for adding another layer of hurt.

"Why?" puzzles and corners feelings. Feelings respond to such questions in a manner resembling having another person ask "Why did you do that?" after we have closed the refrigerator or car door on our finger. Attempting to answer the question logically does not take away the pain, but it can stimulate us to become angry. Anger is a form of hurt. Now, we have two hurts to deal with and resolve, as opposed to the original one.

Other writers acknowledge the misapplication of posing "Why?" questions when attempting to explore and resolve feelings. Emotions are experienced at varying intensities at different times. Often they are felt long before logical rationales surface. They may appear solo or among a mixture of other emotions with whom they coincide or conflict. "Why's?" result in intellectual exercises in rationalizing excuses for feelings, while avoiding means for their resolution.

In the example of the client with the contracted elbow discussed previously: "Why's?" may lead him to the awareness he harbored anger towards his mother. However, he would still be left without workable how-to's for resolving the anger to achieve sustained, longer-lasting relief from the stressful emotion.

Rather than quizzing with "Why's?", more appropriate alternatives are to use the words <u>how</u> and <u>what</u>, then proceed to <u>what</u> and <u>when</u>, e.g., "How/What (are) (am) you/I feeling?" Follow later after exploration with "What behaviors can you/I plan to activate for yourself/myself … things you/I can actually DO, to resolve the anger/hurt and release it?" "When will you/I begin to practice them?" Deciding a date and time to begin add commitment to the decision to change.

By further exploring the feeling or sorting, the other person and yourself can arrive at answers to "Why's" listed previously in "Basic Facts About Feelings, #3".

<u>7. Feelings are our natural and most reliable resource for assessing truth and reality.</u>

Emotions work to perform their duties with and without our alert awareness. They gather trustworthy information from several resources—internal happenings and external occurrences. The messages they convey initially announce the impact of their findings upon us, e.g., "this info is emotionally soothing or emotionally disturbing". Though we may not always be aware of the rational justifications for a feeling's arousal at its onset—the answers to "Why am I feeling this way?", since these answers usually come later in the sorting-through process—it is a <u>healthy</u> decision, to:

> pause for a moment
> to consult with our feeling, asking "How am I feeling?"
> before taking action.

Relaxing to flow with feelings allows sorting to ensue—the process of separating the information from feelings and arranging it into a more comprehensible, enlightening and easily-managed format.

8. <u>With awareness or not, every individual stimulates, regulates and terminates each feeling in our own natural and complete set.</u>

Feelings are very private, personal affairs. Their ownership and management are exclusively restricted to the person who experiences them—ourselves.

POWER over our feelings consists primarily of three inherent, inseparable qualities that validate and ensure its presence inside us, one hundred percent of the time:

final AUTHORITY = ultimate ability to make the final decisions regarding our feelings: selecting, regulating and terminating them;

final RESPONSIBILITY = ultimate accountability for decisions concerning our feelings, their course and effects upon us; and

exclusive CONTROL = ultimate or final ability to regulate our feelings from time of stimulation throughout their "stay" or arousal, plus manage the results of their effects upon us.

Just as you imagined, a detailed discussion of personal POWER and its magnificent three components is a box-office attraction coming soon on this tour. Understanding the concept of the uniqueness of our POWER and the blanket permissions it affords its owner is astonishing. It also explains what makes power (with small letters) such a desirable commodity for others to obtain and use for their enjoyment whenever it is perceived to be available. However, genuine POWER (with capital letters) over our attitude is a permanent asset that remains in our exclusive possession for as long as we maintain humanness.

The process towards emotionally balanced living begins with giving ourselves permission to examine the thoughts, feelings and behaviors we employ. We can supportively identify our own areas needing modification and/or change. In time and with practice, we can alter any part of our stress-producing attitude to experience emotional peace more and more frequently.

Modifying old decisions or completely switching to new ones for our attitude involves some amount of change.

*** Please Note As A Caution: before initiating changes in your attitude, it would be beneficial to gather realistic insights into the phenomenon of "Change and the Change Process" and "Grieving"—other fascinating coming attractions during this tour.

Realistic information reduces the amount of fear usually accompanying change. The objective is to assist in preparing for experiences that can possibly occur while moving towards a more healthy and balanced emotional existence.

2. Emotional Programming—Looking Back With Perspective

Feelings, in themselves, are not difficult to comprehend. The status reports and messages they signal to our brain are clear, concise and relatively simple.

Emotions appear complex, baffling and utterly confusing as we begin to attach to a feeling our <u>learned</u> lessons in "How To BE and Function As A Proper PERSON". While growing up, every individual is exposed to a barrage of instructions presented persuasively as fail-proof guidelines for:

> how to think,
> how to feel and
> how to behave.

You will recall from earlier discussions that thoughts, feelings and behaviors form the three basic components of our human attitude.

Lessons are delivered by an assortment of external teachers in our everyday environment. Their primary objective is to acquire and maintain power over us. Included are such authoritative people and institutions as:

family members;

ethnic groups;

peers;

religions;

schools;

jobs (personnel manuals, policies, etc.);

public laws and codes of ethics;

public electronic media: internet, TV, radio, movies;

books, newspapers and other printed materials; etc

The campaigns and pressuring strategies waged by external learning resources upon us to promote adoption of their directives can be quite persuasive. Most of them have existed in some form since the beginning of humanity. Consequently, they are highly organized and sophisticated in methods they use to persuade our decision. Though they cannot achieve realistic POWER over either segment of our attitude, with enough time and dedicated effort, they can succeed in influencing us to accept their guidelines. More often than not, we adopt the externally-defined lessons, or rules for living, as is, unquestioned and uncensored.

Each resource's opinions are accompanied by well-developed, supportive arguments and demonstrations on "correct" ways to think, feel and behave. Upon adoption, their instructions become our pilots issuing directives we have retained internally and continue to follow today. The lessons remain constantly available to use as references for how to manage our attitude and accompany us wherever we go, whatever our activities and involvements. With willing dedication, they stand prepared to relay their formulas for successful living to us at every available opportunity.

Lessons are individually tailored to attract our attention. From experience, outsiders are astutely aware that, in order for adoption of their opinions to occur, they must first, in some manner, attract the target person's attention. Successful strategies used previously include somehow arousing our emotions, particularly fear and anger. These emotions have demonstrated repeatedly to be strong, convincing motivators for promoting adoption of external directives.

Threats are issued to us directly and indirectly, as well as verbally and nonverbally. Promised consequences for refusing to comply to the "Be Scared", "Be Angry" and "I Am Angry" messages may be real, imaginary, previously experienced or unknown.

Often we cling to external opinions or rules for managing our attitude, blissfully depending upon them to be right or flawless, all of the time, "for ever and ever". Adopted lessons are obediently adhered to—or rebelled against—year after year with minimal variation. Corresponding, we sustain the same emotionally stressful feelings year after year as rewards for our devotion. Despite obvious discomforts, the externally-defined lessons, in time, serve as justifications for our present-day attitude.

Some of the information they deliver is rational and feels comfortable when we practice it. Other portions are irrational and use of these pointers result in our emotional dis-at-ease.

Writers have speculated external teachers and their guidelines often misinform us about reality because they neither think nor feel. Regardless of this probability, common sense dictates after centuries of working to persuade human beings, the learning resources are not entirely stupid. They are aware, on some level, without some amount of control over a person's attitude (thoughts, feelings and behaviors), the power and influence they enjoy—as well as their very existence—are precariously threatened.

While external teachers may misinform us, being accurate about their teachings is not their primary focus. Their job is to issue directives—their opinions, based upon their knowledge—accurate, as well as inaccurate. They, too, are struggling for survival and will employ any strategy deemed applicable to maintain their own continuation. Though frequently they purport our welfare and protection are their number one concern, in reality, their uppermost interest is to preserve their own life—to guarantee their own protection—and ultimately to ensure their own preservation.

People maintain the life and health of external learning resources, e.g., society, the civilization. Much of their structure, power and influence upon us are dependent upon the person's CHOICE to accept or reject their viewpoints as guidelines for our own behaviors and involvements.

Opinions advocated by external resources are among a list of options available to us to select from, discard or ignore as we each re-decide. They are not absolutes for achieving emotional health and cannot guarantee emotional comfort simply by obediently complying with them.

You can become aware you have a natural RIGHT and possess the realistic POWER to change former decisions and make different selections of rules to govern your attitude. By doing so, you can be assured of different emotional outcomes to enjoy.

Decisions made previously on which how-to's to adopt for managing our attitude were most often "gut level" or emotional decisions. Consequently, we may or may not readily recall having made them. (NOTE: Strong denials may well indicate you, too, have forgotten). Based upon the information available at the time of our decisions, we selected external directives that appeared to guarantee our survival and simultaneously provide us with the greatest amount of recognition.

People are intuitively aware from birth we require some amount of recognition in order to survive. This is natural knowledge included in the package of being human. It is further substantiated by our characteristic need to mingle with other people occasionally and other living beings and responsive things.

Researchers have also documented repeatedly emotional life is nourished and maintained by recognition. Recognition or attention provides us with confirmation and reassurance we actually exist in space—separate and unique from other persons and things. Whether the recognition received is positive (compliments, smiles, touching, being listened to, etc.) or negative (frowns, put-downs, criticisms, finger-pointing, etc.), it serves to provide us with indisputable proof we, in fact, ARE.

Though positive recognition and approval feel better, negative recognition and disapproval can also maintain our emotional life—however painful it may be.

Intellectually, some of you may nod your head to agree silently or state aloud that, so far, this line of reasoning makes sense. Yet, many people are reluctant to integrate the additional reality—with equal conviction—some portion of our needed quota of recognition, particularly positive recognition, must necessarily flow from SELF to SELF. When this does not occur, we do not develop into healthy, emotionally independent individuals, capable of effectively managing and supporting ourselves emotionally the majority of the time. Instead, we remain stifled in emotional development, appearing helplessly dependent upon others and external things to provide directives to us on "How to FEEL", while constantly hurting.

Unfortunately, while growing up many of us learn to believe the erroneous viewpoint—the "crazy"—declaring positive recognition must come exclusively from resources external to ourselves for it to be significant or valuable. According to rules provided by external learning resources, recognition flowing from SELF to SELF is to be discounted as:

> selfish;
> conceited;
> vain;
> self-centered;
> egotistical;

narcissistic;

arrogant;

narrow-minded;

bragging; etc.

Each label is fashioned to carry a negative connotation directly attached to an unpleasant feeling on stand-by to experience whenever we compliment ourselves and express SELF-love.

In truth, patting ourselves on the back is not all bad. Some amount of egotism or selfish behavior is necessary to grow and function healthily. It re-energizes and refuels our BEING.

You are aware there are extremes to every behavior and the extremes constitute illness and disease. Still, some amount of selfishness is health-producing. This is not foreign information to most people. However, implementing it is often difficult, particularly when we have not given ourselves permission, emotionally, to deliberately practice it.

In addition to being naturally aware we require recognition, we also know, intuitively, most often we recognize or direct our attention to things, events and other people in whom we have some amount of interest and concern.

Whether the interest is inspired from a positive or negative perspective, we simply do not think about nor acknowledge the presence and existence of a person or object in whom we completely lack interest. A complete lack of recognition/attention defines ignoring, a process involving a different set of behaviors. Furthermore, we confirm our interest with positive recognition and approval or negative recognition (put-downs, criticisms, staring with squinted eyes or raised eyebrows, etc), signaling disapproval—whether expressed openly or silently tucked inside our thoughts.

Despite the pressure we feel today to continue to comply, external opinions are not the same as facts. Opinions are opinions and they carry that label to differentiate them from facts. Opinions are flexible and constantly subject to change. By gathering healthy information and practicing the new, over time, formerly adopted unhealthy opinions can be altered. Their survival, duration and power are dependent upon our CHOICE to continue to agree with their premises and practice them.

Conversely, FACTS do not change. They remain consistently true regardless of the influx of information and amount of time. For their survival, they depend only upon themselves and they retain validity regardless of a person's agreement, acceptance and practice.

At times, when we are questioning later in life, some of the rationales we used to select and adopt external guidelines, they can be quite humorous and enlightening. Directives are often delivered without an identified teacher's awareness of messages being gleaned from their behaviors, e.g., non-verbally issued via demonstration, role-modeling, gesturing, etc. As observers, we made interpretations and copied their behavior for our own use.

To illustrate:

> During a personal development class, a young lady relayed while growing up she would often silently watch her mother while she prepared food for cooking. She observed each time her mom prepared a meat roast, she would cut-off both ends before placing it into the roasting pan and it always tasted scrumptious. Therefore, without questioning, she decided this was the correct method for preparing a delicious roast and proceeded to practice this strategy into adulthood.

> Later on a return visit home, she decided to ask her mom why she removed both ends from the roast—knowing the answer would be related to contributing to the taste. Her

mother looked at her and responded, "Because my roasting pan was always too small!"

Regardless of our decision, a healthy response, after examination, is to choose our behaviors because we want to, rather than a pressuring have to, in the interest of our own survival, health and well-BEING.

Choosing to practice or not to practice a behavior from a <u>want</u> <u>to</u> position significantly reduces the amount of emotional pressure and stress that a <u>have</u> <u>to</u> forces us to sustain. "I want to" leads to much more personal comfort in daily emotional living. Though an opinion we use as an attitudinal guideline may have begun as one externally-defined, through personal screening and evaluation, it can be changed into one deliberately and lovingly decided upon for ourselves. While its content may be the same, the pressure exerted by the <u>have</u> <u>to</u> is removed and it is practiced by personal CHOICE.

As stated previously and again if we want to, we own the natural POWER, to alter segments of adopted external directives and to substitute them with preferences of our own. We can also choose to literally turn them off, switch our thinking stations and direct our attention to other matters.

However keep in mind, while making choices for managing our attitude, we are simultaneously selecting consequences or outcomes of those choices. Consequences are the "other half" of choices. In the real world, one does not occur without the other. Still, the RIGHT to choose our own directives is a natural prerogative. With awareness, screening and practice, it can be done healthily and to our own best emotional advantage.

PART II

PERSONAL POWER OVER FEELINGS:
THE MAGNIFICENT THREE

As the curtains rise on-stage, information from earlier presentations provide background stating, feelings are very personal, private affairs. They dwell inside our body as a complete set. In all probability we will not experience each emotion during our lifetime. However, the seeds of each one reside permanently in our core, attentive and ready for activation as needed.

Additional review and for emphasis we repeat:

1) it is impossible to create or destroy emotions. Human capabilities are limited to:
   - stimulating or arousing our feelings to active duty;
   - regulating their intensity and duration once aroused; and
   - shrinking them into returning to at rest or balanced positions again inside us.

   Stimulating, regulating and shrinking abilities are within the realm of realistic POWER we inherently possess over the emotions in our own set. Our personal POWER over them is validated because we also innately own the components of POWER enabling us to perform these feats.

2) Your set of emotions is uniquely separate from mine and every other person's set.

Though there are similarities in how feelings manifest themselves from one person to another, the appearances of your aroused emotions are not identical to arousal of the same feelings in someone else. Even when we participate in the same life event, each of us can experience the same emotion in a dramatically different way (format). We may even react with an entirely dissimilar emotion from the other person. Such variations would not be possible if both sets of feelings were joined or somehow connected to each other.

3) The intrinsic POWER we have over our emotions is also applicable to our own thoughts and behaviors— the two attitudinal partners of emotions.

POWER over our feelings essentially consists of three distinct, yet inseparable properties or segments: AUTHORITY, RESPONSIBILITY and CONTROL—fondly referred to here as "The Magnificent Three". The POWER segments

exist only as a complete set of three,

permanently merged together in perfect union,

literally unable to be separated.

When one segment exists, the other two segments are also present. Neither component can function alone as a separate entity because each depends upon the other two to be realistically operative.

Let's take a look at the components of personal POWER in general, then discuss each in detail.

> AUTHORITY = Declares emphatically ... I ... alone ... have ultimate or final decision-making ability over feelings I experience, including selecting them, deciding their starting point and determining their end-point. It acknowledges: "I select them", "I start them" and "I stop them".

> CONTROL = Underscores ... I ... alone ... have ultimate or final managing and regulating abilities over feelings I experience, regarding their intensity, duration, my responses to them and their results upon me. It boasts: "I regulate the direction of flow and pathway of my emotions inside me".

> RESPONSIBIITY = Validates ... I ... alone ... have ultimate or final accountability for choices I make in feelings I experience. It confirms:

> "Since I select, start, direct the pathway and stop (terminate/shrink) feelings I experience, the end-results are within my jurisdiction and dependent upon me also".

Now think about it for a moment. Possessing all those abilities—that constitutes genuine POWER!!! Read through them again and allow the impact of the information to integrate.

For emphasis we reiterate, the abilities forming personal POWER over our feelings are impossible to disconnect. When exercising our AUTHORITY over ourselves, RESPONSIBILITY and CONTROL are working also. Similarly, if it were possible for, say, RESPONSIBILITY to be absent from us—whether on loan to another person, or idly dangling in space—our AUTHORITY and CONTROL also vacate from us. Absence of either of the three properties would convert us into mindless, helpless creatures, existing much like robots, regulated completely by outside sources!

* (NOTE: From this point forward on the tour, discussions of the three elements of genuine POWER over feelings will be in the format of A-R-C, an easier mnemonic to assist with remembering them.)

** (Reminder: Throughout the tour, words spelled with all capital letters indicate natural and realistic.)

Emotional POWER is individually owned, totally inclusive of all necessary aspects and therefore unlimited—as it pertains to ourselves. This can be quite comforting information. We become aware that, while feelings can become stimulated without our alert attention, once aroused, ultimately they are regulated by their owner.

Initially, we may feel awkward admitting it. However, it is pleasantly reassuring to know, without doubt, we … alone … own the POWER—naturally, exclusively and eternally—enabling us

> at any given time
> to experience any feeling we select
> at any depth or degree of intensity
> for as long or as short a time as we choose.

Therefore, when experiencing an unpleasant feeling, we … alone … permanently possess the POWER over the emotion to interrupt it, sort it out and replace it with any other feeling we choose from among our inherently complete set!

POWER over our own set of feelings is unlimited. We can:

- initiate or stimulate them into active duty;
- inflate them to larger sizes (e.g., deeper depths of intensity);
- cling to them briefly or extensively prolong their stay;
- put them "on-hold"—temporarily—until a later time;
- hide them beneath other superimposed feelings;
- burst their bubble to deflate their strength or intensity;
- clock them out as "off-duty" to shrink them and effectively terminate their current influence; plus
- successfully exchange them for other feelings;

...and much, much more.

However, the extent of our POWER—its effective sphere of influence - is confined to only those feelings we possess, those among our own set. It cannot expand to incorporate another person's POWER over their set of feelings, with or without their permission and attempted donations.

Paraphrasing, just as our POWER cannot fade away because a segment(s) of its composition is missing from us—the abilities are permanent and inseparable teammates—it also cannot expand to annex POWER segments from another person onto ourselves. Regardless of our intent or their accusations, we absolutely cannot acquire genuine POWER over another's thoughts, feelings or behaviors.

The key word here is "genuine". With their permission, and only if ultimately they agree to allow us to do so, we can influence them in making choices for themselves in their attitude. Still, we cannot perform the selection and regulatory tasks for them.

From center stage, let us introduce you to your personal POWER in more depth. Very often during personal development discussions, a clearer explanation of the nature of our inherent POWER led to heightened interest and enthusiasm among participants, along with a willingness to deliberately practice using it.

POWER OF AUTHORITY

Every person innately possesses the POWER of AUTHORITY over their own attitude (thoughts, feelings and behaviors)—individually. AUTHORITY is the ability to make ultimate or concluding decisions for the attitude we practice. Participants during workshop discussions have affirmed that, with or without our alert awareness, we are constantly giving ourselves permission to make final decisions about:

thoughts we entertain,

feelings we experience and

behaviors we practice.

Realistically, there does not exist a resource external to ourselves that is capable of forcing us to think, feel or behave in any manner. At times, admittedly, we may allow outsiders to influence our decisions. But, their ability to influence us is strictly dependent upon our final decision agreeing to allow them to do so. If we decide to object or disagree with the attitudinal choices they urge us to practice, their influence upon us is trashed or curtailed. Their opinions literally cannot infiltrate our final decisions without our permission.

AUTHORITY emphatically and with relief states: "I SELECT IT!", "I START IT!" and "I STOP IT!" These FACTS encompass a complete system.

Think about it! After using our POWER of AUTHORITY to get into a mess of a feeling and being aware our POWER remains permanently inside us ... we own the ability to use the same POWER ... repeatedly ... to halt the feeling we are experiencing. Furthermore, if we choose to, we can exchange that emotion for a more pleasant one to enjoy whenever and wherever we elect to do so. The only person needed to bring about a change in what we are

> entertaining in our thoughts;
> experiencing in our feelings; and
> practicing in our behaviors

is ourselves. Besides, we are the only person realistically capable of successfully achieving these objectives.

More personally, regardless of external strategies used to persuade me to relinquish this POWER over myself, such as:

> opinions, suggestions, advice;
> requests, pleas;
> compliments; flattery,
> threats and other pressure techniques;
> character labels assigned to me;
> bribes; etc …

… it is I who ultimately presses the buttons to stimulate, direct and discontinue practices for my attitude.

It can be comforting to know, without doubt, the opinions, agreements and services of another person, place or thing are not required for us to experience more pleasant feelings. Through exercising PERSONAL CHOICE, we can deliberately take command of our innate AUTHORITY and intentionally make decisions for our return to emotional balance and comfort.

POWER of AUTHORITY confirms the unyielding FACT the emotional distresses and discomforts we live with daily—and their solutions—both begin and end with ourselves alone. The buck starts and ends with decisions we make—and that represents genuine POWER!!

Keep in mind FACTS are not dependent upon our acceptance and agreement to survive and continue. They remain true regardless of changes in our beliefs and fluctuations in our exposures as time proceeds. Realistically, thoughts, feelings and behaviors are subject to final commands of their owner—exclusively. We hire them and fire them at will, merely by making a choice—a decision—to do so.

People have expressed at some point earlier in life, many of us learned to believe the myth purporting we are incapable of making healthy decisions for ourselves to manage our attitude. In essence, we locked ourselves into believing we absolutely have to experience feelings solely according to dictates of outsiders. Like mud stuck onto the sole of a shoe, we attached the unhealthy external teaching onto our natural BEING—our CORE. Subsequently, the reasons for thoughts, emotions and behaviors we practice are assigned or blamed on external authorities, rather than ourselves.

Becoming aware and accepting ownership of our ultimate AUTHORITY, we forfeit these myths depicting us as helpless victims emotionally. We no longer feel obligated to continue using this excuse for SELF-governing. Those who elect to cling to the myth also cling to sustaining tremendous amounts of emotional pressure and stress in daily living.

In retaining the crazy guideline, as we encounter an authoritative person during the course of a day—or one to whom we assign our AUTHORITY—a great deal of time and energy are spent "changing colors". We allow ourselves to be manipulated, continuously altering segments of our attitude each time the other person switches their preferences. Imagine the emotional strain from constantly attempting to assess and please others, then change ourselves accordingly when, say, twenty authoritative people cross our path during a day! It can get to be an exhausting chore and quite emotionally painful after a while.

Without an aware ownership of our AUTHORITY, relaxing to enjoy alone time is virtually impossible. We set ourselves up to experience an increasing intense "need" to be around our assigned authority-figure or someone else at all times. Without their presence and attention (positive and/or negative regard), we feel anxious, lost and insecure. Though our "need" is not realistic, in that the other person's presence is not required for our healthy survival, the feelings it stimulates are authentic. Effectively resolving the feelings necessitate a re-ownership of our own AUTHORITY.

A group of college students expanded here to add another interesting insight. Holding-on to the myth promoting the premise others direct our AUTHORITY can also summon feelings of jealousy and suspiciousness for us to experience—particularly when the other person elects not to be around us. We feel we have to keep them near us constantly and do not trust them away from our presence. In effect, we are striving to be as sure as possible they continue to be attentive to the duty we assigned to them—caretaker(s) of the status of our feelings—in distorted efforts to protect our own feel-goods.

Seemingly it does not matter that, while the outside person is attempting to perform the role of being our authority, simultaneously they are ignoring themselves in achieving their own wants. Though they may willingly accept the task of making attitudinal decisions for us initially, predictably we soon become liabilities to them, rather than assets. Shouldering authority for two people constantly— themselves and us—is not an easy task. In time, the dual job-assignment will become an intolerably painful burden to them they will soon resent.

Suppose for a moment the other person decides to quit their assigned job of functioning as our authority or decision-maker—for whatever their reasons (they grow tired, bored, develop other interests, expire, etc.). What happens to our emotional status? Unless we reclaim our AUTHORITY, our emotional status is left abandoned, precariously dangling in space without an owner and a home—alone, at risk and anxiously hurting. Because we are attempting to disown that segment of our wholeness, we will likely feel compelled to spend time and energies

- attempting to persuade the same person to resume employment;
- searching for another person to hire as a replacement;
- grasping for a stream of other candidates, in the event the second, third and fourth persons quit; etc.

Spending time and energy working to persuade one person or several to take charge of our innate abilities to think and make decisions for the attitude we practice, plus the consequences happily attached and tagging along with their choices, is a hell of a complicated way to spend a lifetime! We have no guarantees their directives to us will be in our best interest. Besides, our time and efforts are uselessly wasted.

In the final wash, we are the only person capable of realistically performing the job of being in-charge of ourselves. As stated previously, there does not exist an external resource capable of forcing us to think, feel or behave in any manner. For an outsider to influence our decisions, we must ultimately decide to agree with their suggestions and opinions. Since our agreement is the necessary factor to even attempt the transfer of power provides evidence of the eternal presence of our genuine POWER of AUTHORITY inside us. In fact, it can never leave us. Activating the final control-buttons for the attitude we practice remains within our personal domain. It has no other option but to continue as our exclusive privilege—for as long as we remain human.

Transplants of realistic POWER are impossible. Believing AUTHORITY over ourselves can be extracted and attached to an outside person or thing is believing in a fantasy. While we may have decided to allow external resources to function as our authority, in reality they remain void of authentic POWER over us.

Pragmatically speaking, they never had it. Legitimate POWER exists only when all three of its parts are present in combination:

TRUE POWER = AUTHORITY + RESPONSIBILITY + CONTROL

Separately and singularly, each segment is as impotent and powerless as auto parts sitting idly on the shelves of auto supply stores. Without its two traveling companions, donations of our AUTHORITY to an outside recipient is "dead weight" for them to carry. Our gift permits them to be "the boss" without the accompanying powers necessary for the role to have significance and impact.

For practice, to alertly regain ownership of your AUTHORITY, state the following phrases aloud to hear yourself saying them:

I give to myself permission …

to choose and make decisions for myself …

in the thoughts, feelings and behaviors I practice …

and I am the only person who can!

In addition to being feasible, the statement is realistic.

While it may feel awkward and uncertain at first to hear ourselves say the words, the words and accompanying emotions feel better and better with practice—through repetition—guaranteed!

POWER OF RESPONSIBILITY

The source or root of the natural POWER every person innately owns over their attitude is our POWER of RESPONSIBILITY. It is the key factor that unlocks the door leading to emotional balance and contentment in daily living. Since it is an inherent ability, it is always present inside us, busily carrying out its functions—with and without our awareness and consent.

RESPONSIBILITY permeates throughout personal POWER where it infiltrates and validates our POWERS of AUTHORITY and CONTROL. It is the fundamental requirement enabling POWER over ourselves to remain energized and effective. Without its essential presence, AUTHORITY and CONTROL become illusions, useless figments of our imagination.

POWER of RESPONSIBILITY functions to substantiate the eternal presence of our abilities to make final decisions at any point in time to:

- choose the content of our attitude;
- regulate the status of content chosen; and
- control the direction and duration of the content.

Most importantly, RESPONSIBILITY ensures or guarantees we play the most significant role in thoughts, feelings and behaviors we live with throughout each day. It authenticates our POWER affirming since we ... alone ... govern all components of our attitude and their activities, we ... alone ... are accountable for results of our choices within ourselves—the consequences of our decisions.

You will recall choices and their consequences are inseparable. In FACT, one does not occur in life without the other cooperatively following. Consequences formulate the other half of choices. Together they demonstrate a basic law of nature: balance. They are naturally, permanently and happily joined together, incapable of existing, one without the other.

You may be wondering, to whom are we accountable? To answer, the executive to whom we are responsible / accountable is ourselves. Though there may be a reluctance to accept genuine SELF-RESPONSIBILITY, it is also uplifting to know, with assurance, your emotional life is in your own hands. It has always been there and it always will be.

Orchestrating and managing our attitude are privileges granted by our Creator to the person hosting the attitude, for use according to our own purposes at that time. Whatever we decide—whether:

> to keep our thoughts, feelings and behaviors as they are;
> to modify them (alter portions of them); or
> to completely change them,

the final CHOICE belongs to the possessor of the attitude. Our emotions are enjoined to assist us in making these decisions by transmitting helpful messages related to happenings occurring in our internal and external worlds.

Despite quantity or the current size of our POWER of RESPONSIBILITY, its seeds are included in our package of permanent human abilities. Additionally, since we know that change, a basic law of nature, is continuous, it has been growing in some direction since our birth, rather than remaining stagnant.

Healthy development of SELF-RESPONSIBILITY is dependent upon exposures to healthy occasions to practice using it. Although some of us did not have sufficient opportunities previously to exercise our muscles in being accountable for ourselves in our attitude, it is never too late to begin practicing.

External guidelines adopted earlier were not always in the best interest of emotional health. Those directives represent someone else's opinions about us and for us—based upon their assessments and centered on their interests. We can take the plunge to listen to ourselves and initiate other more balance-directed options. At least we can begin to try-on behaviors supporting the notion of being a free, SELF-reliant person, capable of making reasonable choices for ourselves.

Accepting RESPONSIBILITY as a unique, positive and endless privilege paves the way for healthy emotional growth. We come to terms with the relieving fact we are using our own POWER, for whatever reasons, to maintain the emotional stress we live with daily—the uncomfortable feelings-consequences of our choices. Conjointly, we become empowered with the awareness that, if we choose to, we can exercise the same POWER to fire former selections, make different choices for guidelines and behaviors, to actively change things around for our benefit.

Continuing to blame others for our knowledge deficits, lacks in experience, teaching us the unhealthy attitudinal guidelines we currently employ ... etc., etc ... are not valid justifications for remaining deficient and repeatedly, obediently adhering to the uncomfortable teachings.

Neither are decisions we made previously for our attitude substantial entitlements for blaming, criticizing and kicking ourselves in the rear-end. Realistically, we do not hurt ourselves emotionally because hurting is fun. Instead, we do so repeatedly because hurting is habit-forming. It can become familiar as the outcome we anticipate enduring. To be pragmatic, if we had known ahead of time—

> before having the opportunity to learn differently, or before discerning positive lessons from our mistakes—

that outcomes of our decisions would be repeated bouts of emotional distress for us, most people would not have continued to practice those options.

Besides, blaming hurts—whether it comes from others or from ourselves. Mauling and labeling ourselves with derogatory name-calling, putdowns, etc., do not resolve unpleasant feelings. Rather, these put-downs pile on additional layers of hurt.

Blaming differs significantly from taking RESPONSIBILITY for ourselves.

Blaming attacks,

while in taking RESPONSIBILITY, we take credit.

Blaming discounts and subtracts from us,

while in taking RESPONSIBILITY, we accept and add to ourselves.

As examples:

BLAMING	TAKING RESPONSIBILITY
"You (I) should have known better!"	"With the additional knowledge I gained from that experience, I can plan changes inside myself to alter outcomes I experience in future similar situations. I do not have to know before I have had opportunity to learn."
"Any fool would have known better than to …!"	"This intelligent fool can learn from that experience. I can choose more emotionally rewarding arrangements of things for myself."

"You (I) ought not to have done that."	"That's one opinion. However, since I had the option to do it that way, I also have the choice to plan another strategy to change results for myself in the future."
"How stupid can you (I) be? Won't you (I) ever learn?"	"I prefer not to condemn myself. Instead, I take full credit for my ability to make my decisions, and appreciate my willingness to risk trusting myself again."

Often when blaming, we tend to mimic or duplicate methods and phrases demonstrated to us by an influential person or resource from our past. We treat ourselves today and others in much the same manner as someone/thing treated us in similar situations previously. The pain we experienced from their blaming differs only in intensity from the pain we inflict upon ourselves today using their techniques. Self-inflicted emotional pain is usually much more cruel and severe.

Our feelings reside within our own jurisdiction and are completely at the mercy of our own jurisprudence. We are the defendant, the plaintiff, the judge and the jury—the total system as designed by our Creator—and whatever we decide to do with our current feelings is our natural prerogative. We cannot be compelled to retain an option selected by an outsider for our attitude—regardless of their pressure tactics for us to comply.

To repeat, POWER of RESPONSIBILITY over our attitude is limited, in that its effective range is confined to ourselves. As in AUTHORITY, it is impossible to expand our POWER to take over RESPONSIBILITY another person owns over the parts of their attitude. In reality, we can be:

> interested in;
> concerned about;
> caring for;
> sensitive to;
> considerate or inconsiderate of; etc.

their thoughts, feelings and behaviors. However we absolutely cannot acquire an operative RESPONSIBILITY for them—regardless of their intentions and our efforts. Neither can they assume genuine RESPONSIBILITY for us.

Accepting RESPONSIBILITY or accountability for ourselves is the key to change. It is the vital link providing the means for emotional growth, its healthy development and emotional peace in daily living.

POWER OF CONTROL

CONTROL is the third component of intrinsic POWER we possess over our attitude.

Authentic CONTROL secures the FACT we retain ... permanently ... the unique abilities to manage and regulate ourselves in the attitude we practice and the results we experience. Along with researchers, numerous people have shared that, when viewed collectively, POWERS over our own attitude permit us ultimately to regulate:

- when our feelings start;
- the growth of feelings inside us, e.g., their intensity and depth;
- the feelings' duration, e.g., how long they last or hang around inflated inside us;
- which body parts to respond to aroused emotions (and possibly used for their storage); and
- how the emotions effect us now and later.

From an earlier discussion during this tour regarding "Basic Facts About Feelings" (Part I: 1.), you will recall once aroused, feelings demand our direct attention/recognition to be effectively resolved, thereby enabling them to return to at rest positions. Positive recognition from us unequivocally feels better to them, rather than ignoring and negative discounts.

Emotions are powerful entities and can work for us or against us. Although feelings are enjoined by our Creator to deliver useful information to our brain, it is the individual who regulates the general nature and specific terms of the relationship feelings enjoy with us. As managers, we ultimately own the genuine POWER ingredient of CONTROL determining whether interactions between ourselves and our feelings will be:

> pleasant or unpleasant,
> cooperative or competitive,
> mutually supportive or
> mutually detrimental.

We have the option to repeatedly sustain emotional turmoil by attempting to assign CONTROL over ourselves to another person. Usually this is done in exchange for the privilege of regulating their set of feelings. With or without the other's permission, we dutifully pledge to nurture and protect their feelings, while harboring the expectation, unrealistically, they will reciprocally do the same for ours—automatically.

Paraphrasing this emotional game-playing maneuver, futilely we work to extract CONTROL from ourselves and declare it the property of an outsider. To fill-in the void created by the extraction, we attempt to extort the other's CONTROL over their set of feelings. Following our unrealistic exchange of controls, we swear by the myth the feelings we experience are caused by the other person. Conjointly we believe, though an honest mistake, we possess genuine POWER to cause their feelings. In essence, we declare ourselves to be automated devices, helplessly dependent, functioning only at the discretion of someone else while expecting them to do likewise.

Believing this myth yields one aspect of the basic contractual set-up for emotional blackmail. (NOTE: Emotional blackmail is discussed in more detail with the emotion "Guilt" later on this tour.).

Usually we do not assign our CONTROL—in any amounts— to others whom we completely distrust or sincerely feel to be incapable of managing us. After all, an assignment to an incompetent outsider is contrary to a basic law of nature: SELF-preservation.

The stress-producing assigning-control process can also be observed in those who practice approval-seeking behavior. Here, we choose to believe an outsider's opinion of us— wherever it falls on the judgment scale that ranges from extremely high to very low—as more accurate than the positive FACTS naturally known by our emotions about us. Seemingly the trusted outsider's viewpoint or opinion is a more valid assessment.

Continuing to relinquish POWER of CONTROL over ourselves is an extremely risky practice and inevitably dangerous to our emotional health. Power is not the type of commodity allowed to dangle around for very long without a claimant. It is a highly attractive, most lucrative, much sought after asset that appetizingly appeals to anyone and everything around—at least for a while, until manipulating us becomes boring and a burden to them.

Still, if you choose to cling to the myth others regulate your attitude, it would be to your advantage to become aware of who or what is pulling your strings. The awareness could well be a beginning step towards turning emotionally troubling circumstances around more in your own favor.

A general mental health point-of-fact that figuratively applies:

When You Choose Not To Be In CONTROL of Yourself,
Someone or Something Else Is!

Realistically, despite the sincerity and intensity of our delegating efforts, genuine POWER to manage, regulate, e.g., CONTROL the emotions in our own set ultimately belongs to the person who experiences them. This natural order will continue as a private, uniquely personal and permanent part of reality, with or without our acceptance and/or approval.

Let's look at the other side of the assigning-control coin. At some point you may find yourself in the presence of another person who is endeavoring to extract your POWER of CONTROL from you for their manipulation. One of the most effective means to thwart their efforts is by setting limits for ourselves. A polite "No, I'd rather not" will suffice, followed by the best rationale or because in existence, "I don't want to", will likely convey your refusal message successfully.

Speaking up straightforwardly for ourselves does not render us insensitive, non-caring, selfish, etc. Instead, it effectively permits the other person who is attempting to control us to know without pretense what we want to do or not do.

Sometimes we elect to function as trash baskets for unpleasant events and emotions being experienced by another person. We permit them to dump their unpleasant feelings onto us, appearing to feel better following, while we attempt to absorb their trash. Afterwards we feel heavy, weighed down and upset. In gesture only, we soak-up their feelings, carry them around, nurture them and attempt to resolve them. With high degrees of skill and accuracy, we can mimic the originator's emotional responses to their living experiences—as though the emotions were our own.

With further examination of the heavy feelings, however, people found transplanted emotions do not belong to them. Feelings cannot leave their original owner. We may imitate the other's responses, but their feelings and their situations remain with them to resolve as they choose for themselves.

As voluntary adoptive carriers for another's emotions, we can change our mind and eliminate the impact their feelings wield upon us. Simply declare the transplanted emotions void of influence over our own daily life. We have the ability and the CHOICE to get the burden of an extra load of uncomfortable feelings completely off our back. Using our innate POWER, we can exercise our options to offer a feeling back to its original owner for their resolution, or leave the feeling dangling in space and up for grabs for some other prospective adoptive host—still unresolved.

Re-owning CONTROL over ourselves emotionally can appear scary and unfair at times. During personal development workshops, there were those who expressed feeling that in re-claiming our CONTROL, someone else will suffer from the loss, therefore we are not taking care of their feelings, e. g., we are not being "our brother's keeper". The scare, however, is unrealistic. Working through those feelings you come to realize you are not injuring nor destroying them or any other external teaching resource. You are merely removing the power they have enjoyed over you. Once you decide to resume ownership of your own CONTROL, you soon become aware the primary fatalities are your old SELF-detrimental, stress-producing beliefs.

POWER of CONTROL completes the circuit of personal abilities composing realistic POWER over our own attitude. Personal POWER is a closed system that continues throughout human life. It guarantees our natural RIGHTS to freedom and wholeness as separate independently-functioning human beings.

PART III

CHANGE AND THE CHANGE PROCESS

Change is a natural, inevitable phenomenon of living. Researchers and daily observations confirm change as the only permanent reality. Nothing and no-one remain the same. We are constantly in a state of flux—continuously moving, shifting and altering our status.

The movement of change is unrestricted. It can flow in a positive and productive direction or take a negative and destructive course. Regardless, it unavoidably continues as a basic and predictable phenomenon of nature.

A person's attitude is included in nature's change process. At times our attitude improves to become an asset to us, while on other occasions it shifts to become a liability to our health status and overall well-being. There are instances when we hold-on to old decisions for our thoughts, feelings and behaviors more vigorously—becoming progressively more adamant about retaining established beliefs and conducts (e.g., "set in our ways")—while at other times we willingly and quickly let-go, replacing the old with new alternatives to try-on for fitness. In either instance, our attitude does not remain precisely the same.

Some people cling to old and established beliefs, feelings and conducts habitually the majority of the time, while others spontaneously release them, letting them go. Repeated practice in clinging to the same old decisions for our attitude or frequently trashing them for new entries, lead to improvements in clinging or trashing, as opposed to maintaining sameness.

To repeat for emphasis, by routinely holding-on, we increasingly improve our ability to remain attached to old attitudinal lessons learned along with our accompanying repetitious responses, moving gradually towards rigidity in our attitude. With sufficient practice, our rate of speed with clinging increases, until it appears to be an automatic response whenever new ideas and information are introduced for us to consider. Most often our behavior is interpreted as resistance to newness and change. However, clinging behaviors are attempts to maintain sameness and the familiar in our daily life experiences. By clinging customarily, unfortunately we simultaneously reduce opportunities to enhance our personal growth.

We regularly resist making changes in our attitude. Instead, old beliefs and conducts are retained long past their constructive benefits to us. Nostalgically, we expect and eventually come to depend upon our old beliefs to be right, flawless and forever applicable to the network of changing experiences in our current life—despite the pain we often recognize and recurrently endure.

After dutifully and obediently adhering to them year after year, with sufficient practice, our chosen external experts on life become the "reasons" we assert for present thoughts, feelings and behaviors—healthy and unhealthy. Common justifications we issue for clinging practices are such statements as:

"That's the way I was raised";

"My mother always said/did .. (or another significant person from our past)";

"I've always thought/felt/behaved that way";

"According to my readings, Napoleon, the Golden Rule ... (or some other authority used to explain our behavior)";

"Everybody does things that way"; etc.

On the surface, such expressions most of us have used occasionally could be interpreted as unwillingness to change. Instead, as workshop participants have acknowledged, underneath the appearance of unwillingness, feelings of anxiety and fear are likely being experienced. These emotions signal the message we lack knowledge concerning trustworthy and workable how-to's for achieving a change towards the better in our emotionally painful status.

The key words here are "trustworthy "and "workable". The title selected for this tour-guide, <u>When Feelings Speak, LISTEN!</u> is pointedly applicable here. You can be assured fear and its decoded messages are going to be discussed in more detail later in Part V.

When changes are implemented rapidly, resistance to them is more severe. Quick changes do not allow ample time needed to adequately prepare ourselves for new and unfamiliar aspects included in change. They deprive us of opportunities:

- to collect trustworthy information about "why's?" and how the changes will proceed;
- to assimilate and integrate new information into our knowledge-base according to our own style of making things make sense; and
- to develop strategies and implement plans for our own emotional protection and security.

Therefore, seemingly as quickly as a reflex, in SELF-defense we may tightly cling to the old until we can collect enough trustworthy information to re-establish our emotional sense of well-being.

Prolonged clinging behavior can become stressful. Without occasionally re-evaluating to update our guidelines or "reasons", the routinely practiced holding-on attitude can grow into SELF-detrimental territory. Predictably, in exchange for using our time, efforts and energies toward clinging, our reward is the same uncomfortable feelings. However, since sameness is impossible, the feelings are experienced as more intense or at slightly greater depths with each episode of practice (e.g., more hurt, greater amounts of fear, etc.). Gradually we become more and more proficient at hurting, feeling scared, etc.

Change means altering our present status and shifting from known, predictable outcomes to unknown and uncertain results. Even when we are aware of our discomforts, let's face it and admit our unpleasant outcomes are not all bad. They really do issue some amount of comfort and security to us. At a minimum, they guarantee, reassuringly, we will continue to experience the same emotional discomforts—a familiar outcome despite the distressing effects.

At the opposite extreme, habitually letting-go of beliefs and responses learned previously, without personal screening and evaluation, is an equally stress-producing practice. This kind of behavior is often seen in rebellion wherein we routinely refuse to follow old lessons and guidelines learned on "How to BE a Proper PERSON" and instead practice behaving directly opposite to them. Rather than thinking for ourselves and making updated, evaluated decisions in our own best interest, the old guidelines persist as our masters, while we behave, seemingly automatically, as obedient mechanical robots—in reverse!

Habitually letting-go conduct frequently leads to feelings of being "lost", insecure, helpless, hopeless, etc. We leave ourselves with little foundation and without direction, floundering through life much like wet spaghetti. We are perceived by ourselves and others as loose, undisciplined, amoral, excessively flexible, "blowing with the wind", etc. These results are just as painful as habitually holding-on.

The key to emotional health is to determine a comfortable balance between the two extremes in behavior.

As related information, people naturally maintain a status of wholeness or completeness as PERSONS throughout our lifetime on all planes of existence. Our completeness includes our healthy parts and areas for improvement. When we decide to make improvements or changes in our attitude, in essence we are choosing to extract an unwanted segment of our attitude from our wholeness to make space for new thoughts, feelings and behaviors. The extraction creates a void or empty space in our wholeness:

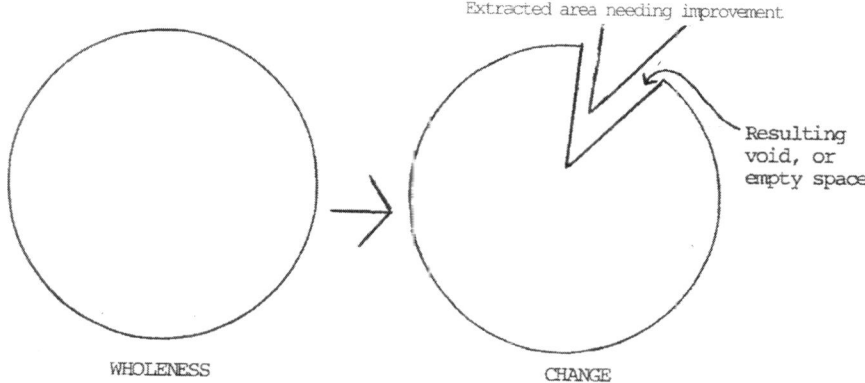

It is a commonly-known fact Mother Nature does not tolerate empty spaces for very long. As voids occur in our physical wholeness, there is an inherent tendency to fill-them-in by shifting surrounding structures; pumping fluids into the vacant areas; developing scar tissue to bridge them; producing more disease tissue; etc.

When we decide to discard unhealthy portions of our attitude and we have not selected healthy replacements, there is a natural tendency for the old and unwanted thoughts, feelings and behaviors to drift back into their familiar, pressuring positions. Consequently, while it is not a have to, we strongly suggest to people to become alertly aware of <u>which</u> healthy practices—specifically identified—we are substituting for extractions before implementing changes in our attitude. Without selecting replacements with awareness, along with a plan of action-steps or how-to's to implement the changes, we will likely resume our downward and painful course of emotional deterioration.

Making changes in our attitude is not always an easy process—even when the changes are personally accepted and wanted. Change means moving from the familiar to the unfamiliar. Collecting information reduces the number of unknown factors involved in change.

While fearful feelings (anxiousness, scared, nervous, etc) signal we lack trustworthy information, with balance as the goal, they are also informing us that, for our own protection, we need to determine practical, step-by-step solutions for problems/obstacles to our attitudinal changes. Many obstacles can be anticipated and workable how-to's for remedying our knowledge deficits can be planned in advance to prepare ourselves in the event those issues occur.

The particular method used to identify possible outcomes of change for ourselves is inconsequential. Available resources to query for suggestions include opinions from other people, personal insights and observations, printed materials, plus speculation, guesswork and pure fantasy.

Despite the pain we are experiencing from old beliefs and practices, most people require acceptable solutions to known and/or anticipated problems—things we can, in fact, Do, for our own protection. Specific plans for SELF-protection generally stimulate feelings of security, safety and simultaneously relief from fear.

Change is a multiple-phase process. It involves letting-go and saying goodbyes to the old and familiar and saying hellos to the new and unfamiliar.

To be effective and less traumatic, begin the change process by identifying specifically the thoughts, feelings, behaviors, circumstances, etc. you are releasing (letting-go, saying goodbye to) and those specific others—the new attitudinal practices and their anticipated results you are substituting or saying hello to. Both halves are required steps in the process to maintain emotional balance.

Next, in all fairness, old attitudes previously practiced were not entirely bad—though they were unhealthy and painful for us. They deserve some amount of credit for enabling us to survive until now. Realistically, in their own way, they taught us quite valuable lessons we can continue to use as references on what to avoid for our own benefit.

When saying goodbyes to old attitudinal guidelines and behaviors, acknowledge their positive and negative aspects and give them the credit they have rightfully earned. Since we cannot erase old learning and exposures, in essence we are saying goodbye to the control and influence they had upon us.

As we explore alternate behaviors, it is not absolutely necessary to know with certainty ahead of time which choices among the new behaviors will yield us more and more pleasant feeling-outcomes. Besides, guarantees about the future are impossible to predict. One of the most effective and reliable means for making choices is through practice or "trying them on for size". New options can be practiced in fact or real-life situations and in fantasy, e.g., using our imagination to rehearse the new behaviors in privacy. More practice will be needed once decisions are made.

Keep in mind practice is time-consuming. Therefore, we can reasonably expect becoming adjusted and comfortable with new choices for our attitude will take some amount of time.

Exercising patience with ourselves while developing new skills in SELF-CONTROL is vital and makes the change process easier to accomplish. But do not overly extend the time you allocate for personal pampering. It definitely does not take as long to effectively make changes in our attitude as it has taken to become as we painfully are now.

We can give ourselves permission to delay final decisions until a specific and SELF-determined later time. In doing so, we are giving ourselves:

time to practice new options ;
time to assess their benefits to us; and
time to learn about and appreciate our personal POWER
… throughout the change process.

Designate a specific and reasonable time in the future to decide upon new conducts and another definite time shortly thereafter to assess your progress. Saying "tomorrow" is an unreasonably short length of time, and "later" is indefinite and vague. Both are attempts to sabotage your goal and remain unchanged—as is—and hurting.

Choosing a specific, reasonable time-frame to effect changes in our attitude adds significance to our decisions. It also encourages personal commitment. Commitment is accompanied by belief in ourselves. A combination of these factors—belief in ourselves plus commitment—forms the key to successfully changing our attitude.

<u>GRIEVING</u>

Death is not a limited experience. Wherever change occurs in life, there is death of the familiar. This remains valid whether changes are transpiring externally (e.g., changes in jobs, places of living, sizes of clothes, automobiles, lifestyles, relationships with others, etc.) or internally (personal habits, health status, attitude, relationship with ourselves, etc.).

Realistically, influences enjoyed by our old unhealthy thoughts, feelings and behaviors do not always succumb easily and spontaneously—even when their demise is acceptable to us and wanted. Usually death of their assumed control over us is achieved in steps or degrees. However, on each occasion when a portion of their release is achieved, some amount of grieving ensues. Grieving is the natural sequel or aftermath that follows death.

Fear of death (departure of the old and familiar) and fear of the unknown (uncertainty about the new and unfamiliar) are present to some extent whenever change is suggested. In part, they account for a person's resistance to change.

People actually grieve the loss of old habitually practiced attitude components, e.g., former patterns of thinking, feeling and behaving. The loss may be a negative loss, which is one we agree to discontinue because it no longer has positive benefits for us, but it remains a loss. As such, we will mourn its departure.

The mourning process, however, will not necessarily appear in an easily recognized form. Workshop participants have described their grief with a variety of examples and methods of weeping. Among these are:

> loss of energy, "the blahs";
> unexplainable, spontaneous tears and other forms of crying:
>> (e.g., babbling speech; flushing; excessive swallowing; clearing throat; coughing; trembling; stuttering; pacing; whining; fast breathing; wringing hands; etc.);
> laughing while talking when nothing humorous is occurring or being discussed;
> staring blankly into space;
> flashes of intermittent body chills;
> short periods of depression;
> happy, warm, glowing feelings;
> bursts of extra energy;
> relieving, sudden releases of stored-up pressure, etc.

Some people have even reported feeling as though they were going to die themselves.

Let us hasten to reassure you that You Will Not Die from changing your attitude! It is Death of External Control you are experiencing. The Re-Birth of SELF-CONTROL and PERSONAL CHOICE are occurring simultaneously.

As you proceed in changing portions of your attitude, give yourself permission to take some time to grieve. However, limit the amount of time. Make an aware decision: How long is reasonable and acceptable to me for grieving? Be specific: one hour, one day, two days, etc.

Plan ahead a list of things to do to end the grief period—thoughts and activities that are pleasant to you, with or without requiring another person's presence and participation. Place the list in a convenient place where it can be easily and readily found when needed.

During the time allotted for grieving, practice saying goodbye to the old attitude by stating aloud, so that SELF can hear SELF:

1) what you appreciate about the old attitude (at least it enabled you to survive until now);
2) what you did not appreciate (blocked personal growth; kept you at odds with other significant people in your life; etc.);

3) what you learned about yourself from it that can be useful knowledge in the future (you can make decisions for yourself—after all, you made the final decisions to use that attitude to manage yourself, even though it was unhealthy; you can make plans for yourself; you can follow-through with plans; etc.);

4) what you learned about it from its presence (detrimental effects upon you; created turmoil; etc.);

… then, say "goodbye".

With this process as a guide, we are giving credit to the old attitude for assisting us in surviving emotionally until now. We are also taking credit for the amount of information—accurate or inaccurate—we knew previously that prompted our decisions to adopt those directives.

Following "goodbye", identify specifically those thoughts, feelings and behaviors you are saying "hello" to and thank yourself for re-'evaluating and updating former decisions for your own benefit—steps toward living, rather than merely surviving.

At the end of your <u>planned time</u> for grieving, force yourself to implement some of the items on your fun-list. It can include such activities as:

listening to favorite, soothing music;

dimming the lights and shadow dancing with yourself;

walking outside or going for a drive;

relocating yourself to sit by a swimming pool or body of water;

taking a warm, soothing, relaxing bath (with or without bubbles);

nurturing household plants or outside gardens;

phoning a favorite, supportive friend; or

going to a park or to see a favorite art display.

Regardless of the activity(s) selected, the important point is for you to get sincere pleasure from doing it. They are ways of saying "I love you" directly to yourself.

As human beings, we need to hear and feel expressions of our own affection and appreciation for ourselves directly from ourselves as often as possible. Expressions of SELF-love and SELF-appreciation assist tremendously in making effective changes in our attitude easier to accomplish.

During the attitudinal change process, it is reasonable to expect missteps or slips away from newly selected thoughts, feelings and behaviors, with reversals into practicing the old behaviors—at least on one more occasion. Such slips are not indications we have failed in changing our attitude. As slips are recognized, it is emotionally healthy to

- acknowledge the fact they have occurred;
- apologize to ourselves <u>first</u> and others by our choice;
- forgive ourselves for reverting temporarily;

… then, resume practicing the newly selected behaviors.

Missteps and mistakes are human phenomenon. They are methods our Creator provides for us to learn. Advancing perfectly in any endeavor, particularly emotional growth and development, is an impossible goal to achieve. In the process of learning, human beings make mistakes. Giving up or perseverating (lingering) on mistakes will not correct our original problem-area. It only delays progress in attaining our goals of healthy emotional SELF-management and effective SELF-CONTROL.

As a brief review, to this point we have explored:

1) our emotional level of human living:
    - its composition, permanence and
    - its innate intent to support and assist us in improving the quality of our daily living;

2) fundamental FACTS about emotions collectively, their innate purposes and how they diligently work to carry out their duties;

3) how healthy and unhealthy emotional programming occur:
   - the involvement of external teaching resources;
   - their factual knowledge about our human attitude, plus
   - general preferential methods for influencing us;

4) the basic components of inherent and permanent POWER each person owns over our personal set of feelings, our thoughts and behaviors.

In the event you are considering making changes in your current attitude, supportive discussions were presented to assist in the process. Information regarding the phenomena of change and grieving provide insights that can reasonably be anticipated in advance and recognized should they occur. Our goal is to encourage continuation along the journey through the change process to receive its emotionally gratifying rewards along the way and throughout this lifetime.

Now, the focus will move to identify and explore some common, crazy, stress-producing guidelines people frequently adopt for managing our emotions. Only a few of these popularly practiced directives will be presented. Proven successful strategies or how-to's for making needed behavioral changes regarding these rules are also forthcoming for use as we choose emotional peace and comfort for our daily living.

PART IV

CRAZY THOUGHTS THAT MAINTAIN EMOTIONAL STRESS

People have discussed using similar guidelines to manage their attitude that consensually resulted in emotional distress. We will review several of these offenders and explore their unbalancing effects upon emotional health.

During the review, should you notice a resemblance to rules you currently practice or have heard about from someone else's experiences—it is not required you openly admit it. At the same time, it may be to your benefit to privately update your decisions for using them, in the interest of your emotional balance.

Remember, you have a natural RIGHT to choose among:

> keeping your rules as they are
> > (when done with awareness and understanding the consequences of preferences, this is a healthy decision);
> modifying your rules (making minor changes here and there); or
> completely changing former practices for new personally selected options.

ALL-OR-NOTHING ASSESSMENT SCALE

The All-or-Nothing scale specifies:

> Either achieve All that is expected …
> > by ourselves and others …
> Or take credit for Nothing.

Goals selected,
> tasks and activities performed,
> > relationships entered,
> > > projects undertaken,
> > > > economic levels aspired,

must be totally achieved—as outlined in our own dreams, imaginations and plans or someone else's—or nothing we do towards attaining said objectives can be counted and appreciated.

Applying this scale to measure progress, we set ourselves up to experience uncomfortable feelings. Our attention is severely narrowed to the two and opposite extremes for evaluating our time, energy and efforts: All and Nothing. Factual steps involved in accomplishing any goal are discounted and trashed as though they were irrelevant. In time, they disappear altogether from of our awareness.

What an "ouch!" to impact our emotional level! Intuitively, feelings are aware this method of assessing our progress and that of others is not only unrealistic, but unfair!

This crazy-producing scale pressures us into working diligently to achieve the impossible extreme of perfectly All, while threatening us with absolute failure as the only remaining alternative it supports for appraising our endeavors.

Among people we encountered, not one person readily admitted to sincerely believing life and living can be summarized using these two categories exclusively. Yet, they almost unanimously shared experiencing feelings of frustration, anger, hurt and disappointment (among others) when diligent efforts to achieve All in their doings or activities proved useless.

Conjointly, they had learned the unhealthy directive to merge their identity as a PERSON with their activities. As the result: whenever projects failed, their worth as a PERSON was precariously threatened—e.g., they felt like they were a "nothing's worth of a PERSON". When one declined, so did the other. They had not learned, as yet, how to

- separate their personal identity—
  e.g., their inherent qualities composing SELF as a
  PERSON—
- from their activities and roles.

There is a distinct difference between activities and roles we perform, from who we in fact ARE as a PERSON. Activities and roles demonstrate how we elect to use some of the personal qualities composing who we ARE. Though the two areas of human living are inter-related, they are significantly different groups of FACTS and therefore not the same.

The feelings of frustration, anger, hurt, disappointment, etc. are transmitting messages to our brain the All-or-Nothing method of evaluating ourselves is inaccurate. This is common sense—natural, inherent knowledge contained in our CORE. We are applying pressure to and hurting ourselves by clinging to this crazy belief, thereby jeopardizing our emotional health.

More realistically,
        goals,
                tasks and
                        activities we perform—our Do's—

consist of a series of steps deserving credit individually for contributing to an objective's attainment.

As we readjust our thinking and practice taking credit for each step accomplished, we simultaneously negate even the remote possibility of ranking as "a nothing" in whatever we Do. Among the steps are:

1) Conceiving the idea;
2) Collecting and recalling information related to the idea;
3) Reviewing the information, extracting segments directly applicable to the idea (and discarding the remainder);
4) Developing a plan of action;
5) Assessing potential outcomes of our actions (positive and negative results);
6) Determining solutions to possible problem-areas—in the event they occur;
7) Implementing the plan;
8) Evaluating our progress along the way;
9) Altering the plan as often as needed; and
10) Evaluating end-results including positive and negative outcomes.

The All-or-Nothing scale limits appreciation to the two extremes. Using the well-known percentage scale of 0-100% in analogy, 100 percent equals perfection and zero percent represents failure. From an available 100 options, they occupy only the two extreme end-points and are directly opposite each other on the continuum:

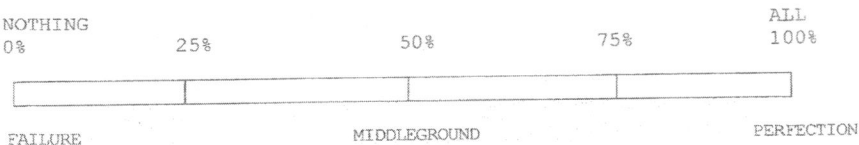

As you can observe, there are no less than ninety-eight (98) additional options existing for describing the stage of our progress—realistic "shades of gray" or middle-ground territory. They, too, are available as choices for measuring our amount of task/goal-achievement ability.

In all fairness, if the only action completed towards accomplishing a goal is conceiving the idea, we are exempt from ranking at zero in ability to achieve the task/goal. Conceiving the idea is a vital activity in the process. After all, without this step the goal itself would not exist!

Feelings and other emotional level phenomena cannot be pressured into limiting themselves neatly into the two extreme positions. Perhaps the All-or-Nothing rule has usefulness on the mental level of human existence, but it definitely does not apply on the emotional level.

Let's return to the popular practice of attempting to stretch the All-or-Nothing scale into a valid measuring tool for determining personal worth. Starting from near the time we were born, most of us learned to believe our personal worth—who we ARE as a PERSON—is the same as activities and roles we perform or what we Do and/or what we Have materially. You've heard the often spoken phrase "you ARE what you Do". The erroneous lessons transmitted herein teach the three categories of daily living as being identical to each other. Realistically, the three are inter-connected, however they are not the same.

Still, people learn this crazy-producing lesson from external teachers in a fashion much like this, as examples:

- New parents bragging proudly to others about how their child ... at two months old ... prepares her/his own peanut butter and jelly sandwiches at the 3:00 AM feeding time. Baby hears this, watches the parents' broad approving smiles and thinks, "I AM a good person because I can Do ....."
- Child goes to school and earns A's for grades. Teachers, parents, everyone proudly pouring accolades upon him/her for repeatedly performing at A-level. Child hears/sees this and thinks, "I AM a good person because I can Do ...." (NOTE : Suppose the child earns a B, C, D or F grade. What value does she/he see SELF as a PERSON then?);

- Person grows up, becomes employed, earns a good salary, has his/her own corner office with a window, big desk, etc. Thinks to him/herself, "I AM an important person because I can Do and I Have …." (NOTE: Suppose he/she gets demoted, office moves to building's basement or they loose the job completely. What quality of a PERSON are they then?); etc.…

As a caution, when your PERSONHOOD is mingled with roles performed (Do's) and/or material items you possess (Haves), your emotional health status is hanging by a thread!

Continuing to cling to the crazy-producing belief the three areas of living are identical, earning less than A's in school feels as though we are a failure as a PERSON; loosing in activities, falling short of expectations in roles performed or loosing a job and we feel, painfully, like a nothing's worth of a PERSON.

Additionally, struggling to apply the All-or-Nothing rule to personal qualities, when we are not using an inherent quality All of the time, as examples,

- confidence, we decide we have No confidence at all; or

- if not feeling secure All of the time, we conclude we are completely insecure; etc.

We negate the innate qualities incorporated in our ESSENCE, refusing to take credit for them in any amounts. Seemingly, those qualities no longer exist as parts of our character description. The reality of their eternal presence—regardless of how frequently we activate them—is ignored.

Usually the wipe-out of ourselves is accompanied by SELF-inflicted, derogatory labeling:

"I'm a non-confident, weak, insecure, dependent, etc. ... type of PERSON"—

additional "ouches" to our feelings and SELF-esteem. Result of our personal put-downs: the unpleasant thoughts and painful feelings we endure multiply!

As we increase our skill in practicing self-annihilation, it becomes easier to recall details of specific incidents almost from birth when, in fact, we were low in confidence, weak, insecure, etc. supporting the negative assessments of ourselves.

When we accept the crazy All-or-Nothing scale as truth, a portion of the hurt we experience stems from inflicting hurt upon ourselves. Intuitively we are aware on our emotional level our positive qualities and personal worth are separate, inherent and forever present throughout our lifetime.

Human qualities are not temporary phenomena, e.g., "here today, gone tomorrow". They are permanent parts of our wholeness. We can CHOOSE to put our amount of a quality on-hold for a time. But, our supply of that quality, regardless of its amount, does not disappear from our essence. It remains available to activate later in other activities, roles and pursuits we select in the future, as we each elect to do so.

To repeat, we own the RIGHT, naturally, to take full, 100 percent credit simply for conceiving an idea—without following-through to a goal's completion. To conceive the idea is a completed accomplishment in itself requiring the use of several qualities from among the extensive list composing who we ARE as a PERSON. In addition, we have the innate RIGHT and CHOICE to be:

> confident when we want …
> weak when we want …
> insecure when we want …
> forgetful when we want …

simply because we want to … at that point in time.

Though we are not capable of showing confidence All of the time, we can take full credit for the amount of confidence (strength, security, knowledge, etc.) we own, even if, in quantity, it equals the diameter of the tip of a pin! That amount of the quality is uniquely ours—one hundred percent of the time—and permits us to rank above the Nothing level in its ownership.

Taking credit for steps toward a goal, plus our inherent human qualities, eliminates the feasibility of ranking as a "nothing" or a "failure" in both areas of our living: Doing and BEING. We have the option to keep performance levels and our amounts of qualities as they are or to increase them, as we elect to do so.

Personal qualities can be increased by pointedly, repeatedly and sincerely summoning them or "calling them up" for active duty more frequently. We summon them up by taking credit for them:

"I AM confident,

I know (for sure) that I AM confident—permanently—

and no one can ... e v e r ... take confidence
away from me!"

Conjointly, we can progress further towards accomplishing a goal by moving on to the next action-step in our goal-achieving process.

BE PERFECT

Now appearing center stage, and linked closely to the All-or-Nothing assessment scale, comes the crazy-producing attitudinal guideline, BE Perfect.

People are born whole, complete with:

> physical body parts;
> a mental or thinking capacity;
> spiritual elements; and
> a complete set of feelings.

As long as some amount of each property is evident, without exception we can be assured of our own perfection. In this sense, perfection is not a matter of becoming or achieving. Human beings who are incomplete as PERSONS simply do not exist.

Growth is continuous. It is a natural indication of the presence of life. In order for it to transpire, some amount of change is mandatory. Throughout growth with its changes, our completeness as a PERSON persists.

Religious scholars attest the original meaning of the term "perfect" was wholeness, e.g., complete with the total package of characteristics differentiating us as human. As time progressed, somehow the interpretation of perfect switched from wholeness to flawless. Flawless is defined as totally without errors and/or areas for improvement.

The switch in meaning of perfect brought with it a twist in how to measure personal value. Rather than beginning analyses of ourselves (and others) from our positive status as a complete PERSON, who changes, external resources instruct us to ignore positives, thereby attempting to subtract them from our wholeness and to use flawless as the guideline for assessing significance as a PERSON.

External teachers enthusiastically promote flawlessness in our character as a feasible goal for human achievement. However, flawless is an ideal and as such, cannot apply to human nature.

Wholeness as a PERSON does not imply we are without flaws. People are born with flaws in every category of our existence. Flaws are underdeveloped areas in our character referred to here as areas for improvement. In addition, people innately possess the unique ability to make mistakes. Mistakes permit learning, growth and expansion to occur.

Reviewing errors we have made can spark such natural freedoms as flexibility, spontaneity and change.

Reviewed objectively, mistakes are not all bad. When permitted, they add to our knowledge. At a minimum, they are valuable references of thoughts, feelings and behaviors used previously that were against or contrary to our overall best interest. Becoming aware of what does not work to our advantage is significant information when updating decisions on behaviors to practice today.

Without areas for improvement and opportunities for learning, further development as a PERSON is squelched. You are boxed-in to the boring cycle of disappointments from repeated attempts to achieve the impossible ideal of perfection, alternated with striving to maintain sameness.

The "BE Perfect/Flawless" standard is an irrational rule for managing our attitude. Rather than becoming flawless, we improve our ability to become rigid and emotionally spent. Perfect people view themselves as finished products. Their thinking is fixed, their feelings formed and their behaviors monotonously boring. For them, life and living loose excitement and appeal. Personal growth, that comes with new learning and exposures, ceases. However, since change is continuous, it becomes apparent after arriving at their assumed "Be Perfect/Flawless" station, remaining there indefinitely to stagnate is impossible. Sadly, the sole avenue remaining unexplored and available to them is rigidity, moving towards emotional death.

Emotional death is more commonly known as insanity—a type of death from which we can recover.

In truth, becoming perfect is an impossible goal to achieve. There will forever be some personal quality, an area of competence, a certain activity we have not yet mastered. After learning one method for conquering mathematics, as example, a new mathematical approach emerges. Once we demonstrate concern with one person using a particular style, another beckons who rejects a similar approach.

There are several disguised, indirect teachings and instructions that promote maintaining the crazy-producing "Be Perfect/Flawless" mandate. Among these are such commonly used phrases as:

> "Do your best";
> "Try harder";
> "Work to your highest potential!"
> "BE a 'good' mother (son, daughter, worker, etc.)"
> "BE the 'most'";
> "BE the 'greatest'";
> "BE the 'favorite'"; etc.

Striving to become the superlative of anything, e.g.,

> descriptions preceded by "most"
> or ending in "-est",

are signals perfection could well be the unrealistic objective. We are expecting ourselves (or others) to make the <u>Guinness Book of World Records,</u> regardless of the extreme in perspective taken—the highest or lowest of that quality.

This is not intended to discourage or disregard a healthy approach to the pursuit of excellence. There are people who experience genuine pleasure from achieving high standards and above average levels of productivity.

However,

> when pleasant feelings occur less frequently and
> our efforts become more labored,
> and compulsively mandatory—
> rather than willing and voluntary—

these are clues "BE Perfect/Flawless" is likely the goal, rather than excellence.

When pursuing excellence, we allow ourselves to have a <u>CHOICE</u> in matters as to:

> when to perform;
> where;
> how long;
> under what conditions; etc

Energy-restoring breaks are permitted also as the need is determined.

If you prefer to cling to some amount of your "Be Perfect/Flawless" guideline, we highly recommend you retain it. However, limit the number of areas for its use and specifically identify those areas. By limiting its use, we significantly reduce the amount of pressure applied to ourselves to perform.

Additionally, specify areas of living and activities you are willing to sacrifice to imperfection—spheres or places where making mistakes are allowed. These become resort areas of living where

> rest, relaxation, and restoration

can transpire. They, too, are necessary to maintain emotional balance.

Recognizing we cannot achieve flawless as a PERSON—a FACT that does not subtract from our wholeness—we can begin learning to accept ourselves for the imperfect creatures we ARE. As human beings, we characteristically possess strong-points and areas for improvement. If desired, we can implement changes toward improvements in whatever areas we select, regulated to our own pace.

The FANTASY in FAILURE

Another connecting link is now entering the spotlight on stage. Most often people who adopt "BE Perfect/Flawless" as a personal goal also experience fear of failure. Failure is the other half of perfection. They travel together as opposites of a balanced team in the natural order of events.

You are aware that balance is a fundamental law of nature. Physics has established for every action in nature, there is a corresponding, equal and opposite reaction: actions and reactions. Failure is the equal and opposite of perfection. Both are outgrowths of the crazy-producing All-or-Nothing grading scale, with the extreme position of perfection representing All and failure providing balance as its equal and extreme opposite. They trek around together producing stress and personal discomfort as a corresponding, inseparable and balanced team. Therefore, positive acceptance of one of these extremes simultaneously carries with it the opposite and negative acceptance or fear of the other:

ALL / NOTHING;

PERFECTION / FAILURE;

Positive acceptance of perfection / Negative acceptance (fear) of failure

In like manner, just as perfection as a human being is impossible to accomplish, failure to be human is equally impossible to score. Our ability to be human is a permanent condition we are stuck with forever—regardless of roles and tasks performed.

External teachers advocate looking exclusively at end-results of activities and performances to determine personal worth. Yet, common sense, our innate intelligence, encourages a more realistic evaluation:

> separate Doings from who we ARE as a PERSON (our BEING)
> and take credit for both, separately, in whatever amounts.

We can practice taking full credit for each step performed in accomplishing a goal/task, along with each quality we use from our personal storehouse to complete each step. In this way, we rule-out the possibility of ranking as a nothing or a failure in both categories. Simultaneously, we can enjoy the feel-goods accompanying taking credit indicating SELF-appreciation and SELF-love—necessary outcomes to maintain emotional health and balance.

Frankly, it is impossible to fail at being human. Qualities and traits composing our humanness, we reiterate, are permanent inclusions in our character. Their eternal presence exempts us from existing as a failure in being a PERSON. While we may fail in achieving external activities, we absolutely cannot fail at being human.

Qualities composing our significance or who we ARE as a PERSON are very different from the tasks we perform. More realistically, we activate qualities from among our inherent assortment to perform activities and roles we select. Human traits or qualities function together enabling us to participate in activities and to perform roles. While the two areas of living are inter-related, they are not identical.

Let's take a look at these categories of living more closely: As example, intelligence is a universal human trait. Every person owns the quality of intelligence simply because we are human. We use some amount of our intelligence in order to:

	think;	eat;
	make decisions;	drive;
ACTIVITIES:	walk;	play;
	talk;	shop; etc.

and additionally as:

	parents;	workers;
	spouses;	citizens;
ROLES:	friends;	students;
	lovers;	writers; etc.

Roles and activities are temporary in nature in that one starts and stops; then another starts and stops; to be replaced by yet another role or activity that starts and later stops. On the contrary, whether we are actively using our amount of intelligence or not, it continues and remains, without fail, as a permanent part of our essence as a PERSON.

Quality or make-up of our intelligence is not the issue here and neither is its source. Whether it be home, street, classroom, or experience acquired, our intelligence remains a constant, continuous part of our BEING. Consequently, it cannot be "lost" or removed from us—voluntarily nor involuntarily.

Quantity or amount is also irrelevant. In amount, our intelligence may be equivalent to a grain of sand. Still, that amount remains ours, one hundred percent. It will continue as a permanent part of each of us for as long as we remain human—whether we intentionally use it or not.

Human traits not actively in use do not disappear from our CORE. Instead, when they are not busy they remain on-hold and resting at minimal levels of activity. They, too, are available for active duty whenever we decide to activate them in other roles and activities throughout our lifetime.

We cannot realistically crown ourselves nor each other as "the best", "the greatest", "the worst", "the least", etc. in any area of daily living. However, our amounts of abilities, as well as our levels of performance, are uniquely ours—a total 100 percent of the time.

Failure and perfection are idealistic concepts and ideals, by their very nature, are impossible to attain. Neither status is applicable to human daily living experiences nor personal traits. Whether we are currently participating in roles and activities or simply being quietly idle and Doing nothing, we remain successful as a PERSON.

We can open the door of availability to our traits by simply acknowledging we have them—alertly claiming them as our own. By repeating aloud a statement such as "I AM intelligent", with pauses between each repetition to feel the statement's impact upon us, we can summon our traits into active duty.

The more positive and direct recognition we sincerely deliver to ourselves—through deliberately, purposefully owning and feeling good about our innate qualities and traits—the more energetic their responses will be as we employ their involvement during endeavors. When SELF-putdown thoughts storm-in to interfere with our ownership sessions—as you can be assured they will do—we can

>   stop the thoughts and
>   put them on hold

until some SELF-designated later time—if ever—using whatever terminology and selection of words that net our halting objective. (Note: Kindly spoken commands are not required to force negative, derogatory thoughts to stop interrupting our taking-credit sessions!)

The choice to discontinue negative disrupting thoughts and to control them lies within the realm of our personal POWER. Negative thoughts cannot continue to interrupt our thinking, feeling and behaving as long as we refuse to entertain them. Just as we can switch radio and television stations at will, we can intentionally change our thoughts to other more SELF-supportive ones, whenever we elect to activate the buttons inside ourselves to do so.

COMPETE AND COMPARE

Approaching center stage for their share of attention is another pair of linked "crazies": compete and compare.

Every goal—realistic or not—has steps leading to its achievement. In compliance, the humanly impossible goals of BE Perfect/Flawless and Failure as a PERSON also have steps promoted by external resources that supposedly ensure their attainment. The crazy-producing steps of compete and compare are used to gauge progress toward perfection and failure.

People in a variety of personal development settings have shared while growing up, unfortunately many of us learn to think primarily in extremes. Using extreme guidelines for measuring, we practice comparing our performances and our innate qualities to those of others.

Often with and without awareness, we decide upon leaders who represent the epitome or model of perfection and/

or failure in a particular activity or personal trait. We then compare their talents to our own performance of that activity and our amount of the same quality. Since we are most familiar with extremes, we make our status assignments accordingly. Regarding personal qualities:

> EITHER: we assign the other person as owning All of the quality or ability, while lowering ourselves to Nothing in that area;

> OR: we inflate ourselves to All, ranking the other person as Nothing.

As example:

> We learn to compare our amount of patience to that of the most patient person we have ever known or heard about. Through comparing, we decide to rank the other person as possessing All patience, while we own zero amount. Whatever amount of the quality we possess is completely nullified from our awareness.

Existing for prolonged periods as a Nothing gets rather boring and painful after a while. In time, to shift from that distressing position, we often compete with our assigned perfect model in a distorted effort to surpass them.

Apparently, the objective in competing is to acquire the coveted crown we assigned to the other person. Having more patience would render to us the one-ups-man-ship status of All—at least temporarily until our next perceived competitor comes along to challenge us for our crown.

Conversely, in rebellion, we elect to be as impatient as possible and to think, feel and behave in manners directly opposite to those of our elected "most patient person". According to our ingenious, though unrealistic scheme, we can become the All in impatience, inconsideration, etc. Regardless of our directional flow—the best or worst in a pursuit or quality—a great deal of time and personal energy are spent searching for perfection (flawless) and failure and striving for their impossible achievement.

Effort by effort, we manage to manipulate ourselves into feeling more and more distressed. Each hurt sustained when we fail to become perfectly all or completely nothing adds to the collection of hurts held in storage inside us. Additional hurts increase the amount of pressure we sustain and in turn sink us deeper into the depths of emotional pain and discomfort.

Perfection and failure are measured by competing and comparing ourselves to others. You can discontinue these crazy-producing practices by simply noticing, realistically, every person inherently owns some amount of the same qualities and abilities in their wholeness just as we possess them. (NOTE: "Yes, but …" responses here are not applicable; plus they are attempts to continue with practicing your emotionally painful efforts to compete and compare.)

Our Creator designed us as separate and uniquely different from each other. Though we have similar structure and abilities, we are not identical. Consequently, it would be reasonable and realistic to presume our universal qualities will vary in amounts from one person to another.

Competing and comparing are emotionally unhealthy gauges and inevitably produce erroneous assessments of personal value. When comparisons are completed and regardless of the tallying scores, other people will retain their amounts of their human qualities, while our amounts will persist as uniquely ours—separately and one hundred percent. Competing and comparing cannot alter these realities.

We can learn to take credit for our qualities as permanent parts of our completeness—in whatever portions and to give credit to others when they demonstrate their inherent quantities of the same traits. These new substitutes in guidelines for managing our attitude have been demonstrated as effective avenues toward emotional balance and comfort in daily living.

BE QUICK and HURRY UP

Rushing now from the left side to center stage is the crazy-producing external mandate to "Be Quick and Hurry Up".

External resources place a great deal of emphasis upon quickness and speed. From almost every aspect of daily living, we are encouraged to adopt quickness as a strategy for healthy human functioning. Living and performing at our own comfortable rhythm are discouraged and often socially forbidden.

We learn to live at rapid paces and with each generation the tempo quickens even more. From every corner we are reminded to:

move faster;

work faster;

think faster;

eat faster;

learn faster;

feel faster;

relax faster;

sleep faster; …

… all under the heading of "progress"!

External teachers predict the quicker and more instantly we perform, the higher we will be regarded, and the better we will feel as a PERSON. They additionally emphasize rewards of positive recognition of our value as a PERSON—pleasant feelings—are conditional, and dependent upon swiftness. Therefore, those of us who are more limited in agility or require more time to complete tasks are to be:

pitied,

put-down,

taken for granted,
and otherwise discounted in human worth.

Well, nonsense!

Daily living experiences repeatedly demonstrate that constantly performing at a rapid pace regularly produces fatigue and often leads to burn-out or emotional exhaustion, rather than pleasant feelings.

Some of us have learned, enterprisingly, to counteract socially-advocated "hurry-up" mandates with several socially-condoned reasons, viewed as justifiable excuses not to perform. External resources have no monopoly on astuteness. People can be quite ingenious in finding acceptable survival-level ways to beat the system.

To relieve some of the pressure from "be quick and hurry up", we may consciously or unknowingly decide to use such temporary and indirect relief measures as:

> physical malfunctions and illness:
>> hypertension; upset stomachs and ulcers; colds; pneumonia; chest pains; joint pains; rashes; headaches; backaches; etc.
>
> mental or thinking disorders:
>> memory loss; inability to concentrate; daydreaming; blocks; forgetting; rambling thoughts; absent-mindedness; indecisiveness; etc.
>
> emotional distresses and discomforts:
>> excessive worrying; prolonged depression; short tempers and angry outbursts; constant confusion; persistent scare; a string of hurts; etc.

Illness is a socially accepted rationale to relinquish "be quick" mandates. It affords time to rest from our labors and permission not to perform. After all, who would dare to require a person who is ill, feeling out of sorts, mentally spaced-out or emotionally upset, to perform, e.g., to do something?!?!

Without doubt, the pain experienced by those who use illness as an escape is real. Such pain is not to be taken lightly nor discounted. More likely however, the illnesses may well be indicative of mental fatigue and emotional exhaustion.

Emotional pain hurts deeply in that it penetrates the very core or essence of our BEING. Yet, it can be more effectively and longer-lastingly relieved as we begin to practice more <u>direct</u> methods for evaluating our current status and discussing uncomfortable feelings to release build-ups of pressure.

Speaking out about our feelings represents only step one in the process of effectively resolving them. Conjointly, with awareness we can select occasions to use our ability to perform quickly and when we will not. We can also plan our time to more SELF-supportively avoid the mandates. Realistically, each of us has twenty-four hours available each day to spend as we choose. How we manage time is an individual decision that also determines the feelings-consequences we endure.

Illness is an effective indirect means for demonstrating displeasure. However, it is temporary and short-term in its problem-resolving effects and personally confining, rather than freeing. Still, we can take credit for selecting and using it as a tool for obtaining some amount of relief from the emotional pain perpetuated by "be quick" mandates. At least, illness assisted us in surviving until the present time.

It would be interesting to survey persons who adhere to "be quick and hurry up" mandates to determine what is the destination. Where are you headed in such a rush? What special treasure waits for you there? Is it really worth the physical, mental, spiritual and emotional turmoil you experience daily to acquire it?

If we are sincere in our desire to achieve emotionally balanced living, it will be necessary to exchange some of the crazy-producing inclusions we have practiced in our thoughts, feelings and behaviors from habitual patterns to different more healthy ones.

> Growth from an unhealthy status
> into a more emotionally comfortable state of affairs
> requires some amount of change.
> To be effective, change requires more time
> in clock hours—
> for practice
> —at least initially.

Common sense teaches when learning unfamiliar things, we literally require more time initially to perform new behaviors and tasks. As we become more familiar with them, through repetition and practice, less deliberate effort and time will be needed. Executing the familiar consumes a smaller quantity of time because, through practice, a lesser amount of change is involved. The new behavior is becoming our newly substituted habit or pattern of performing.

Getting impatient with ourselves while learning a new skill to manage our attitude impedes progress towards emotional health. Plus, it is an attempt, knowingly or not, to hold-on to familiar "be quick and hurry up" mandates and any other unhealthy guideline currently used—though practicing these offenders has recurrently brought us emotional pain.

We have learned to accept quickness as a standard for living despite its unpleasant outcomes. The extreme opposite is to "be slow"—an equally distressing emotional position.

One middle-ground option is to learn how to effectively relax at regular intervals and take restoring breaks. Another is to decide upon a reasonable time-frame, perhaps determined through trial-and-error, we can comfortably follow to achieve a particular attitudinal change.

In the realm of attitudes, the phrase "I can't change" does not apply. Realistically, our attitude is SELF-controlled. Instead of "I can't", the underlying and more sincere message is "I won't", or "I choose not to". You have decided changing is inconvenient for you at this time—for whatever reasons you assign. Therefore, in choosing not to change, you simultaneously elect to retain your feelings-consequences as they are-to-worse.

An insightful speaker once observed principles of banking do not apply to time for happiness. There is no such thing as depositing days and withdrawing them later. If we decide to wait until "a tomorrow" to implement changes in our attitude, on tomorrow we will discover all we hold in our account is a lot of unhappy and exhausted yesterdays.

It would be to our advantage to get off the "be quick" treadmill and to substitute that behavior with our own comfortable, SELF-determined pace. Our pace for comfortably performing is uniquely our own and we will not find another person alive with exactly the same rhythm.

Rather than going through illness and other indirect methods to get permission to slow down, we can consciously, deliberately and directly give to ourselves our own permission. The right time to begin the change is any time—as long as we remain alive and human.

PLEASE OTHERS FIRST—ALWAYS

Strolling onto the stage towards front and center is another well-known "crazy-producer" for display: "Please Others First—Always".

People are by nature social, interactive beings. Intuitively we are aware we require attention or recognition to remain emotionally alive. Getting attention is literally as vital to our survival as are food, air and water. Infants have been known to expire as a result of lack of attention, a condition in crib deaths diagnosed as marasmus. Recognition provides us with indisputable proof and reassurance we, in fact, ARE— we exist in time and space.

Unfortunately, many of us learn to believe we have to depend upon other people for the recognition we require. While growing up we were taught to believe the crazy-producing myth that recognition from outsiders is more valuable than attention directed to SELF from SELF. Adoption of the myth as truth, in effect, assigns outsiders as care-takers of our emotional feel-goods. Therefore, the step we must take, as the myth instructs, to acquire our needed attention, especially positive recognition, is to "please others first—always". Subsequently, we diligently practice this behavior.

Mistakenly, we learn to believe by caring for the interests of "others first—always", somehow we can control their responses to us. After all, we are allowing them, vicariously, to regulate our conduct. In theory only, we donate to others our POWER of AUTHORITY over ourselves (Note: review the previous chapter on Personal POWER), thereby granting them our permission to think and make decisions for us in how we are to behave towards them plus how to feel following our actions. Now, we have set the stage to spend time and energy making every effort to please our care-takers so that, in exchange, they will not instruct us to hurt in some fashion.

People during workshops have expanded upon their experiences revealing very often, we go to extremes to satisfy those others … to get their nods of approval … allowing us to borrow-back our own permission to recognize ourselves—first in a positive manner … at least occasionally … and feel better.

Though some of the strategies expressed during workshops were brilliant for getting attention from others, participants soon recognized they were placing their emotional status in very dangerous positions. Allowing the feelings we experience to be dependent upon the whims of outsiders first, as opposed to our own preferences first, is hazardous business. At best the results are temporary, filled with risks and carry a high probability of jeopardizing our emotional health.

An assortment of explanations for this popular, though unhealthy conduct have been suggested. Among others, fear of rejection, with its threat of aloneness, is frequently cited. In efforts to avoid the guaranteed aloneness predicted and threatened by fear of rejection, we practice going through other people to obtain permissions allowing us to recognize and accept ourselves as a significant, worthwhile PERSON, e.g., to own our own BEING. The permissions we seek include the outsiders' assumed authority over us, on loan to them from us, plus the genuine AUTHORITY over ourselves we are using to re-claim it! (NOTE: An interesting observation here is by employing our genuine AUTHORITY to secure the permission we donated to the outsider indicates the POWER never left us!).

In addition, there is no guarantee the trip through others to get positive attention when we want it will be a gratifying, pleasant journey. The possibility exists they may consent and grant our request. However, unpleasant feelings for us are also available options, particularly when the other person is not in an amicable and complying mood.

Habitual "Please Others First—Always" behavior, by description, simultaneously means "Please SELF Later—

Always". We are pledging to routinely place ourselves on hold until others are comfortable and well-pleased. Obtaining our quota of feel-goods is delayed until some vague and indefinite later time—if ever. Continuing to practice this crazy mandate adds hurts to our internal collection after a while.

Using this stress-producing guideline, the emotional contract with ourselves reads:

> "I agree to put myself off—even if it hurts—while working to keep others emotionally protected, happy and content".

We donate to them our right to feel comfortable and agree, in exchange, to live in emotional pain—a gigantic "OUCH!" to our SELF-esteem.

Others whom we elect to "Please First—Always" have an advantage over us. Rather than controlling them, we are teaching them how to manipulate us. Personally-issued instructions demonstrated by our behavior, inform them how far we are willing to go to obtain their approval. They have the option to require us to complete several tasks before granting our request. Additionally, when we near the completion of one set of their demands,

they can change their mind,
switch their preferences and
issue another series of things to do ...

thereby delaying their approval even longer. There is always the possibility their approval will not be forthcoming—regardless of the regularity and intensity of our efforts to please.

In conjunction with feeling upset with assigned caretakers, some of the emotional pain we endure with "Please Others First—Always" endeavors is signaling the message to us without the outsiders' cooperation, it is impossible to obtain the behaviors from them we desire to feel better. Without their agreement, we can neither control nor manipulate another person's responses. Repeated efforts to win them over add hurts to our own internal collection. Adjunctively, our painful feelings are yelling to us some amount of the hurt we are experiencing stems from devoting too much of our time and efforts to pleasing others, while neglecting ourselves.

Presuming everyone practices "Please Others First—Always" behavior also endangers our emotional status. It exposes us to the unrealistic expectation another person will nurture and care for our feelings during our absence from the job, while we are busily attending to theirs or someone else's.

Despite our brilliant maneuvers, each of us ultimately determines our own thoughts, feelings and behaviors. We may permit outsiders to influence our decisions, but their power over us is limited to influencing alone. Influencing is a process differing significantly from controlling.

Choosing to "Please SELF First—Always" is the extreme opposite of the crazy-producing rule and it is equally as emotionally unhealthy. These are people who fight the guideline by outright defying it and adopting its directly opposite viewpoint, as in rebellion and narcissism. While some amount of selfishness is necessary to maintain emotional health, any activity can be overly practiced. Remember, extremes in any behavior soon constitute disease, accompanied by a variety of disorders in our ability to function throughout daily living.

You may ask here, "Then, how do we achieve emotional balance?" A commonly heard response from everyday people was by consulting with ourselves and activating our PERSONAL CHOICE, we can intentionally decide occasions when we want to "Please Another First" and when we prefer to "Please SELF—First". The decisions become a matter of CHOICE—because we want to, rather than have to.

A tremendous amount of pressure is released by moving from a have to position to a want to stance. The end-results, waiting and available to each of us for experiencing, are commonly known as freedom and SELF-control.

As we begin to initiate changes in habitual practices of "Pleasing Others First—Always" and substituting "Please Others First—by CHOICE", we can reasonably anticipate sparks of resentment and anger from those who benefited from our former behavior. Their unpleasant feelings stem from awareness—on their emotional level—they no longer have the power to control and manipulate us. The amount of their resentment is usually equivalent to the amount of power they felt they owned over us.

It may be helpful to let them know (and to remind ourselves) when we are electing to please them first and when we are not. However, use your own inherent judgment. If you decide to silently retain that information for yourself, in the interest of your own overall well-BEING—though continuing to implement the change in your behavior— that, too, is a healthy decision.

EXTREME WORDS

There are several restricting words and phrases demonstrated to be powerfully persuasive in their ability to control our attitude. They are words whose jobs are to confine our thoughts, feelings and behaviors strictly to the options that include them. Rather than allowing us a CHOICE in matters, they apply pressure to us to recognize and accept the viewpoints containing them as the only correct behaviors available. Most often these viewpoints or opinions (not unyielding FACTS) are ones originally developed by someone and/or something external to us for their own purposes at that time.

The restricting words and phrases have existed since the beginning of humanity and will likely continue in some form forever. Their use is thoroughly integrated throughout our culture. When permitted, they enjoy an increase in their power to unhealthily manipulate us as we repeatedly pressure ourselves with them and/or attempt to exert control over attitudinal choices of others through using them.

Among the list of extreme words that cripple us emotionally are:

> should;
> must;
> have to;
> ought to;
> supposed to;

expected to;

always/never.

At times the words are blatantly used in open statements designed to restrict our thoughts, feelings and behaviors. In other instances, they remain clearly understood communications, though their confining messages are transmitted through such nonverbal strategies as:

tones of voice;

certain eye positions;

facial expressions;

hands on hips;

pointed fingers;

erect body postures; etc.

People learn to believe, unfortunately, by rigidly obeying the shoulds and have-to's—without consulting ourselves for our preferences—magically we will achieve emotional comfort and contentment. Seldom do we accomplish these peaceful objectives. In effect, we disregard our own desires and agree to allow the extreme words to pressure us into conducting our lives according to an outsider's plan.

With enough exposure and practice with the controlling abilities of the words, we become quite proficient in using them. Simply by observing while growing up how people seemingly automatically comply with directives including these extreme words, we soon learn to appreciate the impact of their power and influence upon human behavior.

Through observing and practice, we glean whenever we want another person or ourselves to perform in a particular manner, attaching one or more of these pressuring words to a selected behavior more rapidly secures agreement and compliance. Now we have excellent instruments for stressfully manipulating ourselves and others!

Extreme words are fictitious and impotent in their purported ability to guarantee emotional contentment—our own or anyone else's. They are inappropriate for human thoughts, feelings and behaviors. In the realm of human attitudes, there are no valid or legitimate have-to's, musts, ought-to's, etc. PERSONAL CHOICE dominates instead. In reality, the decision to follow-through with the demands of stress-producing extreme words began with our CHOICE to do so. Conversely, we retain the option to ignore the pressuring words and select the same and other behaviors to practice.

After learning this new information, one workshop participant reported having a sign made and posted in his office stating, "I will not should on myself again!"

For instance, we do not have-to work. We choose to work to enjoy the pleasant and unpleasant outcomes or consequences of our CHOICE. You will recall consequences are the other half of choices, providing balance to the concept.

Among the consequences of electing to work are:

PLEASANT CONSEQUENCES	UNPLEASANT CONSEQUENCES
1. It supports increases in our self-esteem;	1. At times, it is a horrible way to begin a day;
2. It offers a stage to demonstrate our knowledge and skills;	2. We may be required to commit to regular working hours and arriving on time;
3. It provides opportunities to meet and interact with other people;	3. We are required to endure probation and periodic evaluations;
4. It affords opportunities for promotions and career advancements;	4. We encounter some bosses and coworkers with negative attitudes;
5. It awards us money, bonuses, raises;	5. There may be excessive paperwork to shuffle and complete; meetings to attend; etc.

6. It extends to us a company's fringe benefits package (insurances, discounts, off-days ...)

6. We may meet with numerous last-minute deadlines, production quotas; etc.

7. It presents opportunities for professional and personal development; etc.

7. We sacrifice some of our freedom to comply with dress codes; company policies and procedures; codes of ethics; security regulations; etc.

On the other hand, we can choose not to work. Pleasant consequences of our CHOICE include:

permission to sleep late everyday;
more free time;
guilt-free freeloading on relatives and friends;
no conflicts with employers and coworkers; etc.

Unpleasant consequences of our choice include:

eviction;
sleeping on park benches;
going hungry;
repossessions;
fewer items of clothing;
fewer and fewer friends and helping relatives;
jail terms for law violations; etc.

Realistically, people work because we want-to, rather than have-to. The positive benefits of our decision outnumber and outweigh (in value to ourselves) the negative or unpleasant rewards, making the option to work more attractive. In like manner, we can elect not to work. Benefits of that decision are also available to us to experience—pleasant and unpleasant.

Rather than magically resulting in contentment, several participants during workshops reported extreme words endanger emotional health. They contribute additional pressure upon us to select activities and behaviors without screening them through our own preferences and evaluating them for personal advantages and benefits. Those of you who elect to continue to interpret the words as absolutes for managing yourself are also electing to surrender your natural RIGHT to a healthy emotional existence.

Extreme words present their behavioral selections as the singular, most desirable choice at our disposal—the best ways to think, feel and behave. They emphasize an obligation to comply with suggestions they offer inferring refusing to agree is a crime against nature, piggybacked with horrible guilt feelings for us to endure, among other punishments. Our PERSONAL CHOICE is completely disregarded and we are skillfully coerced into forgetting it ever existed.

While the extreme words may ignore our natural RIGHT to CHOOSE for ourselves, it remains eternally operative inside us. To repeat, we exercise our CHOICE on each occasion when we consent to honor the extreme words and follow their instructions for our behavior. PERSONAL CHOICE is an inherent human quality and human qualities are permanent components of our ESSENCE. Consequently, the same ability to CHOOSE utilized then—when we selected the should, have-to and ought-to options—remains a significant and functioning part of us today. We can deliberately activate our natural RIGHT and ability again … repeatedly … whenever we like … as often as we elect to do so.

Choosing how we will think, feel and behave for ourselves are not condemning offenses, but complimentary. The guilt feelings that sometimes follow are, in truth, confirmations we have successfully chosen for ourselves. (NOTE: Healthy interpretations of guilt will follow later on this tour).

Using the extreme words has become a cultural habit that will persist, in all probability, in some format eternally. However, simply using the words does not jeopardize a healthy emotional status. The words, in themselves, do not inherently harbor an element to infringe upon emotional health. The danger exists when we permit the words to exert pressure upon us, demanding we conform to directives they point to. Therefore, rather than squandering time and energies working to eliminate use of the words, a more healthy objective is to:

> redefine them—
> clarifying for ourselves they are not absolutes—
> thereby removing the pressure they apply upon us.

Lifting the restrictions and pressures of shoulds and have-to's permit the freedom and pleasures of want-to's to flow. The want-to's for ourselves may well be identical behaviors formerly mandated by the have-to's—without the pressure!

On a related issue, people with talents in certain areas often feel compelled to exercise our talents whenever needy circumstances occur—though we may actually prefer to abstain. These are persons who learned to believe, as examples:

> because we have a witty sense of humor, we should be the life of a dead party; or
> because we can brew a tasty pot of coffee, we must always be the coffee-maker; or
> because we are talented in mathematics, we are supposed to be the financial book-keeper; etc.

Please be reminded just because it's what you do well does not mean you have to perform the task. Clinging to extreme words forces us into performing because we have-to, rather than want-to.

Eliminating the pressure of extreme words is not achieved by adopting the opposite extremes for our behavior—all-or-nothing. Despite positive intentions, we will again experience emotional distress when we resort to practicing behaviors that are the direct opposite of original "should" mandates. Emotional imbalance will continue as our reward, as examples, when we exchange currently practiced unhealthy rules for their opposite viewpoints, e.g.,

> change from always considerate of others to never considerate;
> move from must work to must not work; or
> switch from ought to, to ought not to; etc.

Instead, lifting the pressure of extreme words opens the door to middle-ground options. It affords permission to utilize our inherent traits and talents wholeheartedly, partially or to keep them on hold—as we decide we want-to about each presenting situation.

In reality, there does not exist another resource with sufficient and accurate knowledge about us to be capable of making decisions on what constitutes appropriate and inappropriate attitudinal behaviors for us to practice. Outside opinions can be useful as references at times, but they remain guesses and speculative opinions on the rights and wrongs for conducts in our attitude.

By assuming AUTHORITY, RESPONSIBILITY and CONTROL over our own attitude, we, too, can arrive at healthy emotional decisions to practice for ourselves.

PERSUADE and CONVINCE

Often people go to great lengths in efforts to persuade and convince others—though the goals are impossible for us to achieve. We conjure up an amazing variety of strategies, angles and schemes to swing another person(s) over to our points of view. To illustrate, in a personal development workshop during a taking credit exercise, in desperation one frustrated group member resorted to offering his partner a ten dollar bribe to change his "I don't believe you" responses he was instructed to say, into agreeing with him while he owned aloud eight of his inherent positive qualities as a PERSON!

The participant explained he perceived his partner's statements of disbelief as legitimate invalidations of his innate WORTH. In addition, he unhealthily:

- assumed responsibility for his partner's disagreement (faulty premise: "I own power over others");
- entertained such self-condemning thoughts as "What's the matter with me?" and "What's wrong with me?" (faulty assumptions);
- declared the opposing opinions as his own fault (faulty conclusion); and
- decided to try harder in his persuasion tactics to correct his errors (useless solutions).

Other people among that group and subsequent groups expressed feeling similarly frustrated with disagreements from others, as well as angry. They shared occasions during their lifetime when, like many other people, they had practiced various sure-shot angles and schemes in determined efforts to change another's opinion, including:

re-explanations, coupled with a seemingly unending series of "becauses";

pleas for sympathy (illness, among other personal problems, attached to justify requests to agree with them);

begging;

threats;

temper-tantrums;

excessive humor;

offering favors in exchange (bribes);
withdrawing to sulk for periods of time; etc

As one strategy proved unsuccessful, they implemented another. Simultaneously, on each occasion one approach failed to achieve the crazy objective—to change their minds—the feeling of frustration recurred, grew more and more intense and moved towards anger.

Using a more balanced perspective, let's take another look at the emotions experienced during persuading and convincing activities. In addition to being painful to us, the uncomfortable feelings of frustration and anger are aroused and on-stage for positive, SELF-supportive purposes. They are working to relay messages to our brain that our goal to change another's opinion is impossible to accomplish:

frustration signals a realistic obstacle is in our path nullifying our power to persuade (obstacle = the other person's preferences for themselves);
anger adds the message we are hurting ourselves by clinging to the myth of owning power over choices someone else selects for themselves.

A recurring explanation for persuading and convincing practices is people often link together several crazy-producing rules for living used to manage our attitude.

We connect the crazies in a chain-like fashion, assuming with their combined strength (energy we have donated to them from our inherent supply of strength), we can more assuredly achieve our impossible goal: to change the minds of others. How ingenious!! Impossible, but clever!

Since many of us have learned, in addition, to measure our personal WORTH according to our performances

when the collective strength strategy also fails to swing
them over—as predictably it will fail—
the depth of our frustration grows, plus
we feel like a "Nothing's-worth of a PERSON.

For instance, we chain together the crazies:

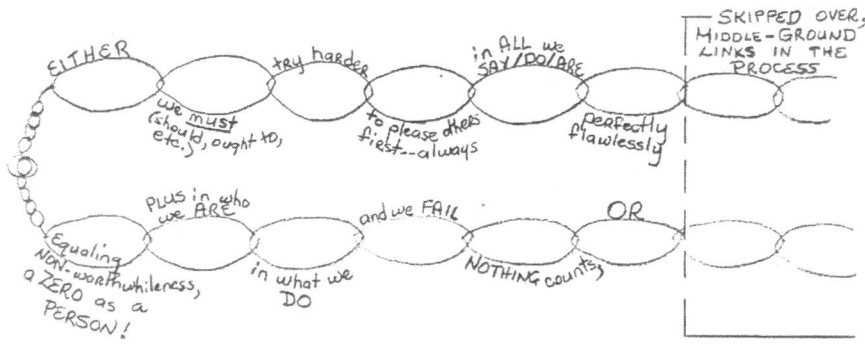

What an amazing twist to reality!!

Regardless of rationales, persuading and convincing behaviors are methods selected to accomplish our crazy objective to control others. More realistically,

CRAZY GUIDELINE $+$ CRAZY GUIDELINE $=$
COMBINED CRAZIES OBJECTIVE

Despite the method of approach ... the extent and sincerity of bargaining and pleading ... and the intensity of efforts ... there does not exist a persuasion tactic nor convincing technique—including brute force and other forms of violence—that can successfully alter another person's prerogatives for their attitude (thoughts, feelings and behaviors). In reality, each of us retains inclusions in our attitude until we individually decide to discontinue them and to substitute them with SELF-selected replacements.

POWER over an attitude is a factual human ability, but it is relevant exclusively to thoughts. feelings and behaviors practiced by ourselves. Similarly, other people permanently own the POWER over their attitude. Just as we cannot donate any amount of our inherent POWER to another, likewise it is impossible to annex a portion of someone else's POWER onto ourselves.

While we cannot persuade and convince another person to change, we can dramatically impact their selections for their behavior when they interact with us. One of the most effective means to influence their choices is by setting limits for ourselves.

In setting limits:

1) Specifically identify behaviors we will no longer tolerate from them.
   For our own clarity and the other person's, narrow generalized, vague dislikes to specific offensive behaviors they practice, plus ...
2) Identify alternate conducts we prefer.
   When requesting another to refrain from a behavior (subtracting), it is vital to also let them know our preferences (adding)—in the interest of balance.
3) State aloud to that person both parts of this message.
   Telling them our preferences eliminates guessing—with its high probability for confusion and incorrect conclusions—while it more assuredly gets for us the behaviors we prefer.
4) Decide upon negative consequences for infringements upon our limits and positive rewards for demonstrations of agreement honoring our request.

Then, follow-through with relevant consequences as infringements and compliances occur.

Perhaps the most significant aspect here is following-through with consequences. Following-through signals interest, concern and respect for ourselves and our well-BEING. It is unrealistic and unfair to expect another person to demonstrate more respect for us than we are willing to practice in our own behalf. The simple truth is we nonverbally teach other people how to treat us by the way we treat ourselves and the permissions we allow them when they are interacting with us and/or around us. Remaining silent when their behavior is offensive encourages them to continue the repulsive practices, rather than squelch them.

Usually, following-through with stated consequences is more difficult when unpleasant consequences are involved. However, when the other person persists with their aggressive behaviors, demonstrating their lack of respect for our emotional welfare, it becomes essential to carry out the pre-selected unpleasant consequences. Despite the discomfort we may experience initially, following-through supports re-education for the other person in how we prefer to be treated and illustrates our sincerity in requesting changes in their behavior. It aligns our words with our actions.

When our words (Say) coincide or match our actions (Do), we demonstrate consistency. Consistency, in turn, confirms for others we are serious about our requests. In time, if they choose to continue relating to us and desire a pleasant exchange, they will also elect to alter their behaviors.

Deciding against following-through on unpleasant consequences, for whatever reasons we assign, gives others our permission to continue their repulsive behaviors. Through our actions we are teaching them our words are meaningless and deserve ignoring. More importantly, in holding-back the consequences, we simultaneously set ourselves up to experience more hurts.

Persuading and convincing are useless, nonproductive behaviors. In the final analysis, after:

> using our time,
> exerting energy to near exhaustion,
> stretching our brain to find new approaches,
> dancing from one effort to another,
> repeatedly tormenting ourselves emotionally, etc.,

others still retain the prerogatives—naturally, permanently and exclusively—to select, manage, retain or relinquish inclusions for their own thoughts, feelings and behaviors for as long or as short a time as they choose.

PART V

DECODING STRESSFUL FEELINGS

AN OVERVIEW TO EMOTIONAL STRESS

Throughout the literature, writers have alluded to emotions as outcomes and reactions to our thoughts and behaviors. Seldom are they discussed directly as important symptoms and clues alerting us to messages they harbor.

Over time in varying personal development settings, ordinary people reported certain consistent trends in information regarding feelings they were experiencing and their interpretations of those emotions. The repetitions sparked our awareness of an inherent knowledge about emotions people hold in common, very likely as a natural part of the package of being human.

Some discussions presented here are supported by other writers. Others may sound familiar to you as we travel, though this presentation is their public debut.

Emotions compose the innate communications system provided by our Creator to keep us connected and accurately informed about our internal world (SELF to SELF) and the external environment (SELF to others). Their primary jobs are to collect information from these resources and transmit messages to our brain for honest consideration and respectful disposition.

Yes, in addition to gathering reliable information, they are enjoined to deliver messages to us pertaining to their findings. Therefore, since delivering information defines a major category of their purposes for existing, our feelings will not rest until this function is also successfully completed.

Realistically, our emotions are our friends. We firmly believe feelings were not permanently integrated into our wholeness by our Creator to work against us in daily living. However, when we disregard their aroused presence and/or ignore the supportive messages they transmit, they do not shirk their responsibilities and obediently return to their balanced and comfortable positions. Instead, emotions grow and expand to yell their messages even louder. Though their original intents are positive, their growth and expansion moves them from SELF-supportive functions into overbearing, SELF-detrimental conducts and results.

The supportive messages harbored by emotions are concise, direct and relatively easy to understand. The information becomes complex and confusing as we attach to our feelings the assortment of crazy-producing lessons and guidelines for living we have learned and adopted from external resources and personal experiences. Several of the crazy-producing guidelines have been presented previously during this tour.

Very often people are not alertly aware of the uncontaminated, simple and reliable information our feelings transmit. While growing up, few of us are exposed to healthy, balanced insights and practical how-to's for interpreting and managing our emotions. Consequently, we wander through life struggling with one emotional upheaval after another and living in constant emotional distress. With enough practice in emotional dis-at-ease, it soon appears to be a way of life and we resign ourselves to the task of adjusting or coping with it—as though distress were the natural order for our daily emotional existence!

The truth, however, is much to the contrary. We do not have to live in persistent emotional turmoil. While uncomfortable feelings cannot be completely eliminated— feelings are permanent parts of our wholeness—they can be healthily and successfully shrunk from overgrown stances into balanced, comfortable proportions.

The process towards regaining emotional balance begins with an alert awareness of new and rekindled information we already intuitively know about feelings and their successful management. As we increase awareness of helpful messages emotions deliver and their unhealthy transmissions, we have opportunity to effectively change our unbalanced, stressful statuses as they occur. We can CHOOSE to update faulty interpretations and practices from those resulting in prolonged emotional distress, into ones culminating in emotional relief and peace, more and more often, throughout everyday living.

With the latter objective in view, let's explore some of the more commonly experienced emotions to collect insights directly from them into the positive and supportive messages they signal, plus some of their negative and unhealthy transmissions once they have overgrown into becoming stressful. While there, we will gather informative how-to's for successfully managing their reduction from overgrowth into returning to peaceful positions inside us.

EXPLORING STRESSFUL FEELINGS

FEAR

Everyone feels afraid some of the time. Perfectly brave human beings do not exist. Fear is one of the most powerful emotions in our innate, permanent and complete set of feelings.

Some amount of fear is healthy and serves useful purposes. Among supportive messages to its owner, fear signals we:

lack trustworthy information;
lack preparation; and
lack protection.

However, as we collect more trustworthy information, we become better prepared and can more capably plan for our own protection. The end-result is a reduction or shrinkage of fear.

Fear is one of the largest emotional cripplers and killers known to humanity. It thrives on assigned power and control and will enterprisingly scheme deceptive methods to exploit its owner when allowed.

Fundamentally, there are four categories of fear:

> fear of the unknown;
> fear of death/change;
> fear of rejection (being found out, aloneness); and
> fear of failure/success.

These may be experienced separately or linked to each other in a chain-like fashion.

Occasionally we allow extra amounts of fear to live inside us for a time as a source of additional motivation and alertness. Far too frequently, however, we permit the excess fear to overstay its welcome and to remain long past its productive and beneficial limits. Consequently, it is important to take some time to re-evaluate our fear and determine when it has become unhealthy and counter-productive.

Numerous people have shared excessive fear has several unhealthy or negative purposes and effects:

- it keeps us immobilized, frozen or locked into a particular viewpoint or frame of mind;
- it sabotages us and keeps us from getting our real wants;
- it bluffs us into believing it to be our protection, urging us to hold-on to it, thereby lengthening its own overgrown status and life style of power and control over us;
- it campaigns for adoption of the "others first—always" guideline coupled with threats of an impending loss; warnings of loneliness; reminders of our weaknesses; reviews of our errors made previously; etc.;
- it doubtfully questions our ability to successfully manage and protect ourselves by suggesting a variety of negative potential outcomes and "you can't make it" messages. The intent is to sell us a 100% guarantee things cannot work out in our favor as long as we are in charge of the CONTROL over ourselves.

At initial inquiry, deceptive and overgrown fear cleverly describes itself as our protection. Among its distorted messages is underneath its supposed protective shield resides additional scares steaming-up from a horrible monster known as SELF. Fear's intention, offered convincingly, is to protect us from discovering the beast.

Deceptive fear continues, claiming it protects us by preventing others and ourselves from finding out about our soft or weak spots. Our hurt from that disclosure, it predicts, would be too great. In addition, others will automatically become our persecutors. Fear reasons without it to protect us, we would be left vulnerable, helpless and defenseless—a state absolutely certain to result in more emotional pain.

Recall for a moment the sorting process advanced for exploring feelings presented in "Part I:1. Basic Facts About Feelings, # 5—# 6" of this tour. The sorting process continues here by posing and answering for yourself the following inquiries. Remember to refrain from asking "Why?" questions.

> How am I feeling? Answer: scared, fearful
> When did it start?
> What was going on?
> Who was there?
> What was happening and what was said?
> How did I hear (interpret) these actions and what was said?
> What is my fear telling me positively?

> Answer: I lack trustworthy information—
> I lack preparation for myself—
> I lack protection for myself
> How can I fill these voids so I can feel less fearful?
> ***Develop and implement a plan of action!

Upon exploring the emotion in more depth, people soon became alertly aware, in reality, our sources of strength, realistic SELF-protection and POWER over our fear are stored within the alleged beast—ourselves. They are integral parts of the positives we inherently possess as a human being. Rather than protection, our overgrown fear is serving as a block to prevent us from becoming aware of our innate positives and alertly enjoying their presence.

Deceptive fear keeps our positives hidden, concealed from our own awareness and unable to be observed by others. As opposed to our strengths, we and others perceive only the fear. Both parties are reluctant to approach us and establish closeness. To them, it seems smarter to keep away from us, in the interest of their own safety and well-BEING.

The resulting double-bind or "can't win" position manufactured by excessive fear, in fact, guarantees our aloneness, hurt and rejection. Emotionally, we are left stranded someplace, having been deserted by ourselves and others. We consistently deny ourselves permission to develop close relationships with ourselves and other people, leaving fear as the only remaining companion for us—gloating in its power and control, while gradually growing in strength and vitality.

Realistic outcomes of fear's purported protection are total aloneness, extreme hurt and complete rejection. However, when we continue to agree to refrain from re-evaluating our fear, it has ample time and opportunity to expand and increase in assigned power over us.

Deceptive fear's goal is indeed protection, but not for the individual experiencing it. Its true goal is to protect itself, beginning with sustaining its own life style with more donations of our power to use in controlling us. It is keenly aware it can only attain power over people who perceive themselves as helpless and hopeless, doubting our:

> ability to trust ourselves to collect reliable information;
> ability to learn in order to get prepared; and
> ability to protect ourselves emotionally and otherwise.

We have lost sight of our innate POWER over ourselves, leaving the job of managing our POWER vacant and available for fear to grab!

Offers of power are reputably desirable and pursued items. Seldom, if ever, can power be found lying idly around without a manager attached to it. People and things gobble-up power at every opportunity. Therefore, you can be assured whenever we are not in charge of the POWER over ourselves, someone or something else is.

Power offerings are of number one, top priority interest to fear because it absolutely cannot grow without our power donations. Without our contributions, fear is doomed to living as a suggestion to us concerning our deficiencies, rather than a controlling force.

When we sincerely decide to discontinue or fire fear as our manager, and re-own our innate POWER, the negative outcomes predicted by fear can be valuable information. We can use them to plan the attitude and activities we will practice, beginning now and into the future, in the event the forecasts occur—thus shrinking our overgrown fear. Strategies for SELF-protection can be developed from fear's projections as our first step towards implementing change. They can also be used to determine detours toward our goal of SELF-CONTROL. In these ways, fear's negative presumptions become useful, beneficial suggestions to us in collecting trustworthy information, as opposed to deterrents to SELF-improvement and/or goal achievement.

For practice in shrinking fear, divide a sheet of paper into two columns. In one column, list fear's predicted negative outcomes, beginning with the worst possible event that can occur and proceed to the least fearful possibility. Let your imagination flow. In the second column, list solutions to each outcome—things you can actually implement (Do) to take care of yourself if the projected outcome happens.

PREDICTIONS OF FEAR	SOLUTIONS
1) (Worse fear) _____	1) If this happens, I will Do _____ for myself.
2) _____	2) If this happens, I will Do _____ for myself.
3) _____	3) If this happens, I will Do _____ for myself.
4) _____	4) If this happens, I will Do _____ for myself.
5) (Least fear) _____	5) If this happens, I will Do _____ for myself.

Then, review your chart as often as you like. We can make our mistakes on paper, rather than living through them. Conjointly, we are assembling and organizing information for our own preparation and protection. In doing so, we simultaneously release the grasp of fear and reclaim POWER over ourselves that fear has vicariously enjoyed.

At times, fear can mask or cover excitement. We get to the brink of achieving our goal—a much desired want selected by SELF—and fear steps in to prevent us from completing the task and feeling successful. Fear can present success as a painful experience, scaring us with threats of seemingly justifiable reasons to avoid it. In truth, successfully achieving our wants demonstrate the inaccuracy of fear's predictions and rob fear of its power to unhealthily manipulate us.

At the opposite extreme, failure is usually perceived and experienced as repulsive and intolerable. Countless hours are spent and enormous energy with continuous efforts attending to minute details to produce a perfectly flawless product or result and indirectly to feel like a success as a PERSON.

Very often, we mistakenly practice equating our performances, (our projects/ products), material possessions and ourselves as a PERSON, as though they were one unit—the same. This is particularly apparent when we have not been exposed to the opportunity to learn realistic differences among these three aspects of our human existence. As yet, we are not aware that, while these three categories of living are interrelated, they are not identical.

(NOTE: Take a moment to review the process for separating our BEING from Doing and Having as advanced previously on this tour in "Part III: Crazy Thoughts That Maintain Emotional Stress": "All-Or-Nothing Assessment Scale", "BE Perfect" and "the Fantasy in Failure"). Be assured, while our activities or performances may not win academy awards, and the products of our efforts may be flops, we can never fail at being a PERSON.

During personal development sessions, various participants expressed fears of success and failure as borrowed scares on loan or adopted from an influential person or event encountered in their life. Among reasons issued for denial of their success and repeated failures were veiled warnings and threats gleaned from these external resources assuring an inability to achieve successes in general, and guaranteeing their failure.

On a feelings level, like gum stuck to the bottom of a theatre seat, the sharers had attached the crazy messages to their CORE. Thereafter, the "you'll never make it" or "you can't make it" messages were used as valid predictors of their endeavors. In many instances, the unfavorable outcomes were pertinent to the outsider's life experiences and were being mirrored to scare, sabotage and prevent participants from enjoying their share of successes. Duplicating the outsider's experiences with failure was made to appear to be a safer route, with predictable feelings-outcomes, rather than stretching into the new territory of success.

In this instance,

the opinions and experiences of another become All,

- while positive factual qualities intuitively known about ourselves, plus
- healthy pleasant steps toward goal achievement during experiences in our past—

become Nothing.

With excessive fear's encouragement, we manage to nullify legitimate reasons for achieving goals in distorted attempts to protect ourselves and the other person from experiencing the overwhelmingly uncomfortable pains of success. Our time and energy are directed toward avoiding success to preserve another's image and protect the unhealthy relationship we have established with them.

Let us digress momentarily to reassure you becoming aware of crazy-producing words and messages used to govern your attitude previously until this time does not imply we have to (have to = crazy extreme word) overtly confront external teachers and resources to persuade (persuade = crazy extreme word) them to change. Convincing them to change is not the objective here! (convince = crazy extreme word)

Becoming aware offers us opportunity to modify or change crazy-producing directives housed on our feelings or gut level and halt the powerful impact these unhealthy messages have wielded over us. Yes, without doubt, we eternally own the ability and the POWER to remove the fallacious blob of gum stuck on the bottom of our theatre seat, e.g., our CORE.

The objective here is to reclaim genuine POWER over ourselves, effecting more pleasant and less emotionally-stressful living—daily—for ourselves. However, when we change our responses to crazy lessons learned and start enjoying successes we have earned, the other person will likely change positively also to some extent—if they desire to continue relating to us.

To continue:

Fear will assign All or total responsibility to us for protecting the integrity and personal esteem of others, as though they were helplessly incapable of performing these jobs for themselves. It also threatens rejection and aloneness if we elect to change how we function in a relationship that is emotionally draining for us, while the other person enjoys emotional contentment. By agreeing with fear's rationales and following its instructions, simultaneously we set ourselves up to fail.

Keep uppermost in mind this reality: If they choose not to alter their practices in discounting success, you cannot change their opinions until they agree to permit you to influence their decisions. Authentic POWER over their attitude remains with them eternally. It cannot be manipulated, exchanged, etc.—just as our Creator intended.

Conversely, in rebellious fear of failure, we work towards making the other person's warnings and negative opinions about us, plus their successes and failures to equal the Nothing. Fear of failure is used to motivate us to become All and to guarantee our arrival at that station. Devotedly we cling to fear, diligently striving for flawless activities and projects, expecting ultimately to feel like and become flawless as a PERSON. Through-out the expenditure of time and efforts, we deny ourselves the natural RIGHT to be successfully human.

In reality, earthlings such as human beings have flaws inherently, and characteristically possess the ability and freedom to make mistakes. Flaws are positive components of our character. They permit opportunities for growth to continue, while mistakes contain avenues for learning. Through objectively reviewing mistakes, we can learn how to avoid the same types of failures in current and future endeavors.

Just so you will know, the purposes of excessive, deceptive fear are:

> to immobilize us;
> to demonstrate our inability to accomplish goals; and
> to distract us from reality.

There were members among the workshop groups who expressed having difficulty recalling a time in their lives when they did not feel afraid. To them, seemingly there had never been such a fear-free time. They have held-on to fear for so long, it has become a way of life.

For them, living without fear feels like an unknown. The only evidence they have such a lifestyle is possible comes from observing other people who demonstrate fear-free living. Changing their own lifestyle, however, to one without fear's heightened companionship feels quite risky. Without doubt, they can anticipate little if any cooperation from power-hungry fear to voluntarily shrink to assist in the person's efforts toward change.

The very notion of changing to a different way of living triggers another category of scares: fear of death. Fear and SELF have coexisted for so long eliminating one is equated, on a feelings level, with eliminating both. In addition, fear of the unknown and fear of death will link together coordinating their strengths to prevent initiating changes in the lifestyle we agreed upon with fear to establish and retain—regardless of the amount of discomfort and pain we experience. Unhealthily, we agree to cling to fear providing it with a happy home, while fear agrees to keep us "protected" using scare and isolation.

Let us hasten to reassure you that you will not die from making changes in your thoughts, feelings and behaviors—your attitude. It is death of control by fear and death of the unhealthy-but-familiar outcomes that we experience during change. The re-birth or re-ownership of SELF-CONTROL and PERSONAL CHOICE occur simultaneously—very natural and healthy substitutions for our losses readily available to us for enjoying.

Excessive fear does not remain static or stationary. It, too, changes in dimensions just as other phenomena in nature. When permitted, it grows and expands, becoming more intense and generating pressure. The pressure exerted by prolonged clinging to excessive fear gets very heavy and difficult to sustain after a while.

Very often, after holding-on to feeling scared for a time and continuously ignoring its supportive messages, we experience fear's frequent traveling companion—panic. Panic is one means nature provides to short-circuit or interrupt prolonged periods of feeling afraid. While it offers some small amount of temporary relief from persistent nagging fear, panic does not afford a long-lasting solution to removing or shrinking fear's grasp.

Panic episodes are popularly referred to as "going crazy", "freaking out", "clicking off", "snapping", etc. They are examples of temporary insanity and, as such, are forms of emotional suicide—a type of death from which one can recover. Consequently, our ultimate negative reward or unpleasant benefit, experienced in exchange for clinging to fear indefinitely, is outbursts of crazy behavior.

In most instances, panic episodes are guilt-free in that the person feels no remorse about their bizarre behavior. They have later explained the panic episode as though it were a positive, asserting they were not responsible for themselves during that time. Unfortunately, in the course of events, believing we can occasionally lack POWER over ourselves (genuine AUTHORITY, RESPONSIBILITY and CONTROL) becomes acceptable to them—at least temporarily.

Realistically, however, people habitually hold-on to uncomfortable feelings for the secondary benefits they yield. Some of the benefits or rewards for clinging to being afraid are:

- we do not have to change, but can remain in our uncomfortable, shaky ruts;
- we do not have to confront new and uncomfortable situations (someone else will do it for us);
- we can get some amount of positive recognition from rescuers;
- we can continue to appear helplessly immobilized, making no further independent decisions for ourselves;
- it is an effective method for controlling others, as long as they are willing to believe we are helpless;
- it is an excellent excuse for blaming an external resource for our mistakes and misfortunes.

If you are a person who has allowed fear to control you for whatever reasons, for whatever length of time, here is a healthy suggestion:

> rather than condemning yourself for using fear, compliment yourself!

You found a creative means for surviving emotionally to the present time. Looking back objectively, its selection may not have been to your optimum advantage, but fear has helped you to survive until now. With information available to you during earlier years, choosing fear to control yourself seemed to be the right thing to do. However, with new information as you are presently collecting, you can regain and sustain your own innate POWER with awareness and alertly practice exercising your own CONTROL over yourself.

Reprimanding ourselves for our lack of knowledge about an issue before having opportunity to learn about it, hurts and adds to our discomfort. Rather than discounting yourself with such labels as coward, chicken, ridiculous, no guts, etc., use your time, energy and effort to educate yourself and to practice SELF-CONTROL of SELF.

Remember, the learning resources in our environment, for the most part, neither support nor condemn a person's sanity, comfort and balanced emotional living. They merely state their positions and opinions. If you had known in the past the natural knowledge you are rekindling now, you probably would not have selected fear to control you. Forgive yourself, then decide to change your attitude to live the remainder of your life less traumatically.

We have the natural RIGHT, the POWER and the CHOICE to benefit from knowledge attained from living under fear's shadow. At the least, we learned how to live miserably. We can choose to change original decisions and to select other means for living that are more to our overall benefit as a PERSON. The CHOICE to do so, however, is ours—individually.

Caution:

When you decide to implement plans to relieve yourselves of excess fear, you can anticipate experiencing some amount of grief. You may recall from a previous discussion, grieving occurs whenever there is a loss—whether the loss is a positive or negative one for us—and it can take on a variety of appearances. It may be beneficial to briefly review the discussions on "Change and the Change Process" and "Grieving" presented previously on this tour to assist in preparing for making changes in your current emotional status.

ANGER AND HURT

Anger is a very powerful motivator of human attitudes. When aroused, it demonstrates a tremendous ability to influence the conduct of our thoughts, feelings and behaviors throughout daily living. Like other emotions in our inherently complete set, anger has positive and supportive messages to us for consideration, as well as negative and detrimental transmissions.

From its healthy perspective, anger is our natural internal barometer signaling personal hurt.

ANGER = HURT.

Hurt expressed outwardly is known and recognized as anger. When our outbursts occur, everything and everyone near us can easily identify our presenting emotion as anger. On the other hand, when we swallow our hurt and retain it inside, it exerts its angry attacks internally and is known as depression. Therefore, the primary difference between anger and depression is the direction of our expressions of hurt.

Guidelines for living taught by external resources promote the fallacy instructing by ignoring our hurts, somehow they magically evaporate and disappear. Not only is this mythical belief untrue, it is misleading. Once uncomfortable feelings are aroused from their at-rest positions, they have a message to deliver and do not tolerate being ignored or flipped-off.

Refusing to acknowledge the presence of our anger and, more significantly, deciding against resolving the underlying hurt directly that it signals will not eliminate the hurt. The pain will still be expressed in some manner. Rather than evaporating, the hurt directs itself into an internal compartment somewhere inside us where it joins other shrugged-off hurts. Each ineffectively resolved hurt adds to the stock we harbor in storage. While in storage, their restless activity continues.

You are aware from personal experiences anger is not a cool, calm type of emotion. On the contrary, it is quite active and hot. Its constant activity resembles a covered pot of water placed on a flame and coming to a boil. In time, pressure will forcibly escape from the top of the covered pot to intrude upon surrounding structures.

In similar fashion, anger restlessly churns. The heat and turbulence of its movements are observed through such behaviors as

hostile voice tones—raised or barely audible;
pronounced body gestures;
clenched teeth and fists;
firmly held lips;
protruding neck veins;
flared nostrils;
facial frowns;
crying;
profuse perspiration;
tightly squinted or blazing eyes;
increased heart rate, pulse beat, respirations and blood pressure;
slumped shoulders; etc.

When the feeling is left ineffectively resolved, its hot, churning activity generates energy and build-ups of pressure. In essence, anger will build to a point of explosion and splatter onto anyone and anything around. Explosive overflows, however, do not resolve the collection of hurts. They merely allow for more space within the pot or temporary relief, until the internal pressure again builds to explosion level.

Hurt has external and correlating internal expressions. Increases in amounts or heights of anger have similar internal expressions corresponding to increases in depths of depression. To illustrate:

HURT EXPRESSED EXTERNALLY (ANGER)	HURT EXPRESSED INTERNALLY (DEPRESSION)
"ticked off"	"the blahs"
irritated	some loss of energy; decrease/increase in appetite;
upset	disinterest in environment and people around us;
mad	socially withdrawn; isolated;
irate, violent	strong feelings of helplessness and hopelessness;
homicidal	suicidal

Left ineffectively resolved, anger and depression can increase to extremely painful and potentially lethal emotional proportions. Homicidal and suicidal feelings are indicative of huge quantities of personal hurt.

Realistically, feeling as though we want to eliminate someone else or ourselves is not the same as doing so. We can feel like we want to kill, but having the feeling is very different from performing the act. The feelings of homicide and suicide are among our natural and complete set of emotions. As warranted, they are available to each of us. While experiencing the feelings is not a crime, a sin, etc., following through with the actions are misdeeds. Still, few people serve jail terms or offend our Creator because we experience the feelings. Such consequences are reserved for carrying through with the destructive actions.

Once aroused from its peaceful position, anger demands direct attention from its owner to complete delivery of its supportive message that we are hurting. With extended presence, the feeling is experienced as though it were in charge of us, instead of SELF in control of the emotion. The longer we attempt to ignore our hurt, the more it grows and the more pressure it exerts upon our entire existence to be heard.

Excessive anger is quite versatile and vicious. It can attack us

> physically to:
> > freeze itself in body joints;
> > rip into internal organs;
> > erupt our skin surfaces; etc.
> mentally to:
> > infect our thinking processes;
> > block memory;
> > disrupt concentration;
> > scatter thoughts;
> emotionally to:
> > make us supersensitive and paranoid with "chips" on our shoulders;
> > carry us through a roller coaster of uncomfortable feelings; etc
> spiritually to:
> > stimulate distrust in our abilities;

    lower self-esteem;

    encourage disbelief in a Superior Being; etc.

To be pragmatic, people can be very creative with indirect methods of expressing anger/hurt. Short of exploding in anger or becoming deeply depressed, knowingly or not, we practice roundabout or disguised ways to demonstrate our anger. We may have learned to seal our lips, ignore the angers and pretend nothing has happened. Ironically, however, the pressure we exert to keep a hurt feeling sealed inside also permits it to escape or slip through our facade to display itself anyway.

Intentionally or intuitively, we usually learn another person's likes and dislikes—the "do's" and "don't's" they endorse for their own comfortable living. When we get angry with those persons, we zero-in on performing some of their "don't's".

Admittedly, using indirect methods to express anger may relieve our hurt feelings temporarily, though their effectiveness is short-lasting. The feelings will inadvertently resurface in similar situations at a later time. We may forget details surrounding anger-provoking events occurring in the past. But, the feelings experienced on those occasions, when ineffectively resolved, remain alive and active. Left unattended, they resurface whenever similarly painful situations occur today. In the present time, those old hurts are popularly referred to as our soft spots or weak spots.

Regardless of its appearance, pathway, manner of expression, etc.,

> anger directs its primary operations and
> exerts its maximum effects
> upon the person who is hosting it—SELF.

While we in error practice assigning the blame for our emotion to an external source (e.g., "Jim made me angry"), the principle victim of our anger is ourselves. We suffer the unpleasant consequences for recent hurts and our excessive amounts held in storage.

The primary purpose of a person's anger is to supportively alert its owner we are hurting and neglecting to soothe our own emotional pain. We have agreed with an outsider's unfavorable opinion and/or demeanor concerning us and joined them in negatively attacking our ESSENCE. Neither of us is showing compassion towards SELF.

Legitimately speaking, another person's (thing's) viewpoint cannot hurt us unless we agree with their negative opinion, then we follow-through to negate the positive, permanent FACTS we intuitively know about ourselves.

Some amount of the hurt we sustain results from neglecting to take positive credit for ourselves. Hurt is the price we pay for overlooking our emotional protection and failing to nurture ourselves among our list of things to do. Others can support us in personal soothing efforts, but they cannot pull the strings of genuine CONTROL governing our feelings to relieve hurts on our behalf. That job or ultimate POWER belongs exclusively to us—individually—just as our Creator intended.

Rather than lingering indefinitely on the anger, let's begin working towards emotional healing by focusing attention on our hurt. As one lady during a personal development class eloquently related, when we experience anger or recognize it in others, a healthy, aware and supportive response could be:

> "I hear/see your anger, but I know you are hurting. How can I help you?"

In actual situations, we usually have trouble initially narrowing-down to identify specifically what hurts. It is less difficult to recall the sequence of events and behaviors provoking our anger. Discussing details of an anger-provoking circumstance is healthy and often necessary to ventilate the emotion, e.g., air-it-out before we can arrive at specifics about what are our hurts. However, limit the amount of time allocated to ventilating. Next, identify what is painful about that issue with questions and answers to include:

> Is the accusation true about me?
>> Answer = No, then drop it and turn the page!
>> Answer = Yes: Where did that idea about me come from (in the past)?
>> What is the evidence of its presence today? (present)
>> Do I want to change that about myself? (future)

If change is desired, develop a plan and implement it. If not, for whatever reasons you assign, deliberately inform yourself of the same knowing you will likely suffer similar uncomfortable outcomes in the future. Sincere responses to these questions can lead to longer-lasting emotional comfort.

A second method, particularly if you find after honestly answering the above questions you are still having trouble letting go of your anger, take a future trip. Answer for yourself:

> "If I decide to continue to feel this amount or intensity of anger through the next week, what effects will it have upon me and my ability to function:"

for the next month?

for the next three months?

for the next six months?

for the next complete year?

for the next two, three, five years? etc.

Proceed in time as far as you prefer.

When you arrive at the end-point of tolerance for your anger, look back through time to today. Now ask yourself:

"Since I have a CHOICE in the matter,

do I really want to spend the next five days (weeks, months, years)

experiencing the same boring angry feelings

and living with the same-to-worse results

OR

would I prefer using my time and energy in other ways more

pleasant and beneficial for myself?"

Regardless of your responses, you are making a decision to use in managing your attitude. That CHOICE is your RIGHT and prerogative to make. Remember, the outcomes we experience and live with daily are controlled by our own CHOICES.

Openly acknowledging anger and hurt to an offending person face-to-face is not an absolute necessity. We can imagine or pretend their presence, seat them across from us and ventilate our anger towards them with equal effectiveness. However, if you decide to directly confront an offending person, own the feeling you are experiencing as yours. As examples:

"I felt angry (hurt) when you ____"
as opposed to, "You made me angry when you ____"

Owning the feeling reduces the other person's immediate need to defend themselves. They may be more willing to listen to us, rather than impulsively reacting in retaliation or self-defense.

Whether we choose the face-to-face approach or fantasy, disclosing our angry and hurt feelings represent only one-half of our responsibility in this exchange. To briefly review:

- We have identified the offending events and/or behaviors we feel warrant our anger (hurt);
- We have expressed the anger as our own ("I feel angry ....").

The remaining part of the process continues with:

- informing them of our preferences for their behavior towards us in the future:
"Rather than doing/saying＿＿＿, I would appreciate you saying (behaving) in this manner towards me instead (continue with your preference)".

Set limits for ourselves, including positive consequences for their agreements and negatives for infractions, along with a commitment to ourselves to follow-through with said consequences

first, for our own emotional balance and comfort—and theirs secondly—by our CHOICE.

Stating solely what we dislike about another's words/behaviors/activities is incomplete. It merely lets them know a problem exists. By adding our preferred alternatives—as suggestions for their consideration—we are providing them with workable solutions. It eliminates guessing games and incorrect assumptions, conserves their time and effort and more assuredly gets us what we want in their behaviors.

Keep in mind the other person also has choices. If they elect to continue the offensive behavior, a significant message is there for us. It would be to our advantage to explore the behavior with them as to:

its meaning or intentional message;
its duration (how long they intend to continue it); and
their expectation of us in how we are to respond to them.

When we decide to release our excessive anger, we can reasonably anticipate some amount of grief. Though the loss is a negative loss or one to our benefit, it remains a loss. As such, we will likely grieve its departure. Allowing ourselves time for grieving is healthy, but limit the time. At the end of that time period, say goodbye to your anger/hurt and move on to live the remainder of your life less painfully.

DEPRESSION

Depression is anger directed internally rather than externally. Anger, in turn, is our innate signal alerting personal hurt. Therefore, depression is another emotion noting the presence of personal hurt:

DEPRESSION = ANGER = HURT.

During workshops, respondents reported in this culture people learn the outward expression of emotional upsets is socially unacceptable behavior. However, keeping angers and hurts corked inside is condoned. We are taught to believe, unfortunately, our primary duty in life is to protect the emotional status of others. Additionally, we assume everyone practices "others first—always" behavior and therefore, eventually, our favors toward others will be returned to us—automatically—by some other care-taker. Meanwhile, we leave ourselves emotionally expectant, but unprotected and hurting.

We cling to these emotionally unhealthy lessons and use them day after day in managing our attitude. We diligently work to refrain from openly expressing angers/hurts—even when they begin as small irritations—and instead strive to pretend they do not exist. Resembling a cork placed in the neck of a bottle, we seal aroused angers/hurts inside and instruct ourselves to ignore their presence. Society teaches the more we practice this concealment process, the better we will feel and the higher we will be regarded as one who "maintains control".

Feelings, however, do not conduct themselves according to the same socially-taught standards for living. Nature's laws governing activities of our emotions were developed by their

Creator—a Resource far more Superior and Sophisticated than mankind and our everyday society.

Once our emotions are aroused from their comfortable positions, they do not obediently subside and disappear.

> When we do not acknowledge the presence of our anger—
> even if confessed to no other person but ourselves—
> and we refuse to hear its supportive message of personal hurt—
>> rather than shrinking,
>> the feeling grows
>> into a deeper depth of depression!

The hot churning movements of a larger amount of sealed-in anger apply even more pressure to internal structures surrounding it.

On the emotional level, our feelings instinctively register the information we are practicing the crazy-producing socially taught rules and building-up pressure inside. Corking angers internally to maintain control requires a great deal of energy and it is personally painful rather than pleasant. Emotions on-the-scene are doing their job to observe what is happening and collecting information regarding events within our internal world from SELF to SELF. They experience the pain resulting from our practices and intuitively know that

to silently and angrily wait
—indefinitely—
for someone or something external to us

to change their attitude (thoughts, feelings and behaviors) from neglecting, abusing, being inconsiderate, etc. of us, into becoming more respectful and nurturing toward us
is painful

—particularly when the external other does not have the same desire for themselves, whatever their reasons.

While waiting for the outsider to change and corking-in more and more anger on each occasion they do not, we, too, neglect ourselves. As opposed to implementing pre-planned activities to nurture and soothe our own hurts, we mimic the outsider's behavior and overlook ourselves also. In essence, we have assigned total responsibility for resolution of our hurts to an external person/thing—a choice filled with risks, yielding a high probability of additional hurts to endure.

Realistically, a portion of the anger we feel is with ourselves. We are hurting by refusing to attend to and protect ourselves. One method of bringing our attention to this painful predicament is by issuing the message to our brain, via our feeling of depression, that in addition to permitting outsiders to infringe upon us, through personal neglect we are assaulting ourselves. Whether we do not know how to nurture ourselves or we do not care about ourselves, the fact remains we are not protecting and taking care of the person who is our primary responsibility—ourselves. Frankly, our aroused and angrily depressed emotion does not appreciate the situation.

For a moment, imagine a bottle without a cork in its neck. The movement of air flows freely from inside to outside. As fluid forms (hurts), it is released or evaporated, preventing the opportunity for build-ups of pressure to occur.

The uncorked bottle represents the person who realistically is "in-control". These are persons who:

- acknowledge the presence of anger/hurt to ourselves—first (fluid in the bottle);
- take time to determine what happened (from another and ourselves) to prompt the feeling's stimulation;
- develop and implement an action-plan—e.g., Do something to release internal pressure from

ourselves, ideally as it occurs while it is small … to feel better. (NOTE: addressing hurts need to occur at any time—whether they have grown into a huge proportion or remain small.)

Our action-plan may include one or all of the following:

- admit our anger/hurt to ourselves, along with becauses;
- express our anger/hurt to the offending person— directly or in fantasy; and/or
- make an aware decision to Do nothing at the present time for our protection—though we may know the whys and becauses for our anger/hurt. However, still plan a specific future time to re-evaluate this choice.

Regardless of the option selected, use your innate judgment to make an aware decision regarding which available action(s) will likely net you the greatest advantage(s) at the time or in the near future.

Some amount of internal pressure is naturally released with each step completed in the problem-resolution process. Regarding the management of emotions, we are not required to wait for relief until the final step in the action-plan is accomplished and the votes are counted. Nature is not that cruel. Rather than draining our energy and wasting time, futilely, to "maintain" emotional control, our energy is available for redirecting to other issues in living.

Depression has also been described by personal development participants as the distance between what we want and/or expect and what we, in fact, have. The greater the space between these two factors, the deeper our depression:

$$\frac{WANT/EXPECT}{HAVE}$$

To illustrate: if what we want is companionship, but what we have is aloneness, we experience depression.

Holding-on to the want,
dangling it teasingly in front of ourselves,
but electing to continue to remain isolated
from other people,
the distance between the two factors increases,
and our depression grows to a greater depth.

On the other hand,

> as we begin mingling and interacting with others,
> in search of a friend, lover, etc.,—
> and take credit for each step taken towards this want
> or goal—
> the distance between the two factors lessens.

Correspondingly, the amount or intensity of our depression shrinks. Finding that special other permits our want and have to merge, e.g., space between the two factors is no longer present. At that point, our depression related to that issue is reduced inside us to its balanced position of calmness and peace.

When our goal requires only ourselves, we can achieve it nearing 100 percent of the time. The only person required to obtain the want is SELF. However, when it involves another person and/or thing, the realistic possibility of acquiring the goal is reduced, with responsibility for it distributed among the number of subjects involved. Successfully attaining the want is contingent upon another person(s)'/ thing(s)' agreement to cooperate with us—usually with some secondary benefit for themselves.

Suppose our want depends predominantly upon another person, and their choice for themselves differs. Frankly, we cannot achieve our desired objective. A want for another person or from another person, when they disagree with that desire for themselves, is an impossible goal for us to attain. As examples:

- Wanting attention from another person, while they staunchly refuse to comply yields lack of attention for us from that person. The lack for us will continue to be a reality, as long as the other person retains the same decision for their behavior (want from other);
- Wanting another person to clean-up their language in public (want for other) as a display of respect for themselves, etc., while the other person harbors no desire to do so—regardless of consequences for them—yields continued rotten language from them. That reality will persist as long as the other person maintains the same choice for their behavior.

Continuing to cling to impossible wants add to the quantities of anger/hurt we harbor and constitute personal set-ups to experience depression.

Many times verbalized wants vary widely from our behavior. People often talk about desiring things to be different, but we continue devoting time and efforts to practicing decisions to the contrary. Intellectually, we rationalize with an assortment of seemingly justifiable reasons or excuses for not working towards achieving goals—whether with altering our attitude, living circumstances, etc.—in efforts to substantiate and retain our current depression.

In actuality, the identified goals lack commitment of our time and energy with follow-through behaviors confirming our movement toward achieving the expressed goals. As a realistic rule of thumb, truth is evident when there is consistency or agreement between our words and actions:

TRUTH: Say = Do.

Spending time practicing behaviors contrary to verbalized wants or our Say, makes the words become dishonest:

UNTRUTH: Say ≠ Do.

The inconsistency demonstrates us working against ourselves.

This is not intended as a discount to our purported wants. It is an awareness necessary before attempting to make re-evaluated, updated decisions for the attitude we will practice, beginning today. If you choose to retain the want, it would be beneficial to place it in a more realistic perspective. The want remains real, but we choose not to allocate time and energy toward attaining it at the present time—for whatever reasons. When this decision is made with awareness, it is a healthy decision and negates excuses for remaining depressed.

Additionally, in selecting wants for ourselves it is vital for choices to be realistic and attainable. As discussed previously, wants for and from other people/things are conditional and dependent upon the other's agreement and cooperation.

Even when our wants require mainly our own efforts and participation, it remains important for them to be realistic and attainable. Therefore, upon deducing, as example, we cannot become a pilot as aspired, before feeling more depressed, another helpful process is in order:

> separate the meaning or significance of the goal (task, role, performance, material possession—our Do's and Haves's)

> from the goal itself.

Then, proceed to selecting other avenues to give to ourselves those same or similar meanings under another label, job-title, activity, role, etc.

WANTED JOB: Pilot

MEANINGS TO
MYSELF

1. feeling powerful and in-charge
2. freedom to make decisions
3. status/prestige
4. increased self-esteem
5. indicative of high level of intelligence ("smarts")
6. attractive uniforms to wear
7. higher paying salary, etc.

ALTERNATE JOBS
AVAILABLE

1. aviation comptroller
2. accident/incident/investigator
3. business personnel manager
4. independent business person
5. policeman/fireman/paramedic
6. community leader/organizer
7. captain of sports team, etc.

In this way, we allow ourselves the pleasures of achieving the significances piloting offers—the underlying core reasons for selecting the want in the first place—via an alternate or back-up plan of action. As one participant in a personal development class insightfully observed:

same objective, different route.

Malicious depression can attack our entire existence with much the same vigor as excessive overt anger. Meantime, while we busily spend time feeling depressed, it greedily collects our strength and vitality for its own survival and grows!

Keep in mind, depression can only acquire power and control over those of us who perceive ourselves as helpless and hopeless. Still, even from these positions, we have abundant reserves of strength. The same energy and POWER we theoretically donated to our depression, in fact, never left us. Such transplants of realistic POWER are impossible to accomplish. We have merely been directing our POWER to service our depression, rather than ourselves.

Genuine POWER over our own attitude (ultimate AUTHORITY, RESPONSIBILITY and CONTROL over our own thoughts, feelings and behaviors) is a permanent part of each of us for as long as we are human. We eternally reserve the natural RIGHT and prerogative to use it with awareness … repeatedly … for our own benefits and to re-claim it at any time towards feeling better.

Rather than abandoning ourselves, leaving us emotionally unprotected and feeling empty as a PERSON, decide to learn how to give to yourself restoring fill-ups. Others can support us in developing the new skill, but the job remains ours to perform. With a sincere desire to shrink our depression, we can achieve this goal.

We have the choice to hold-on to our amount of depression for as long as we prefer and maintain the distance between what we want and what we have. On the other hand, we can redirect our attention to closing the gap, and journey towards emotional peace. The process begins by taking credit for what we have now—in whatever amounts— in relation to a goal's achievement. In addition, we can make changes and substitutions in our own attitude in SELF-selected areas as we deem necessary and at our own comfortable pace. Conjointly, since we are the persons who are hurting, as signaled by our depression, we can learn:

- to forgive ourselves for mistakes in following-through;
- how to nurture ourselves—at least some of the time; and
- assure achievement of some of our wants during this lifetime.

As we sincerely decide to surrender portions of our depression, we will likely experience some amount of grief—particularly when depression has co-existed with us for a prolonged time-period. Giving-up its constant companionship is healthy behavior, but it constitutes a loss and as such we will grieve its departure.

It is helpful to recognize the grief for what it is and to give ourselves permission to flow through it. However, set a reasonable time-limit for grieving. Additionally, since grief can assume a variety of forms, it may be useful to review the sections of this tour on "Change and the Change Process" and "Grieving" to interpret your experiences in shrinking your depression more healthily.

GUILT

Some amount of guilt is healthy and contributes positively to our overall emotional status. Like fellow emotions among our innately complete set, guilt's primary purposes are to collect information and deliver messages to our awareness for respectful consideration. Though its intrinsic intent is to be helpful to us in daily living, most of us have learned to perceive guilt feelings as punitive—emotional penalties for:

> wrongdoings performed;
> mistakes made;
> crimes committed; etc.

in our thinking, feeling and behaving. Using these negative interpretations as guidelines, the emotion is experienced as a chastisement, rather than a support.

Among its healthy messages, constructive guilt is our internal signal alerting us:

- we are <u>not</u> attempting to assume or take-charge of responsibility (accountability) for someone/thing else—whether for their thoughts, feelings, behaviors nor the resulting outcomes they experience; and
- we are successful in our efforts to "put ourselves—first", healthily, on a particular occasion.

Relinquishing endeavors to take-on responsibility for another person's attitudinal components is healthy behavior to practice. In addition, "pleasing ourselves—first" some of the time maintains our own emotional balance. To support our constructive behavior, guilt feelings let us know we are on the right track towards these emotionally beneficial goals.

Perhaps the most pervasive and irrational themes promoted by external resources as appropriate guidelines for managing our attitude are other-responsibility and SELF-sacrifice. These themes are particularly prevalent in feelings of punitive guilt. Outsiders strongly recommend adoption of the irrational themes because they provide steps or how-to's toward achieving the stress-producing mandate to "please others first—always" in our daily living.

Let's take a closer look at these two absurd themes.

Crazy-Producing Theme # 1: Assume Responsibility (small letters) for Others

To briefly review from an earlier discussion during this tour, every human being comes equipped from birth with genuine POWER over our attitude and outcomes we sustain resulting from our choices. Each person's POWER is permanent and separate from every other person's POWER over their attitude—just as our Creator intended.

Realistic personal POWER consists primarily of three components or abilities that absolutely cannot be disconnected one from the other: AUTHORITY, RESPONSIBILITY and CONTROL. Whenever POWER is operative, all three elements must necessarily be present and functioning together as a team in a unified effort. Isolated and alone, each component is as useless and ineffective as owning electrical appliances without electricity.

Despite these FACTS, external teachers begin early in our lives promoting the fallacious premise that we have the ability to remove another person's/thing's authentic POWER of RESPONSIBILITY from them and graft it, magically, onto ourselves.

During rare moments when they choose to be truthful, external teachers may fleetingly admit the POWER we possess over our attitude is a permanently owned package of abilities, thoroughly integrated into our human essence. Obviously, they may shrug to add, an outsider cannot actually push our buttons forcing our final decisions to start and stop practices we select for our own attitude—our POWER of AUTHORITY. Neither can they regulate the content nor the directional flow of thoughts, feelings and behaviors we experience—our POWER of CONTROL.

Parenthetically, just so you will know,

- decisions others make to agree with our suggestions for their behaviors do not validate our ability to manipulate some segment of their attitude; and
- when others follow/reject our advise, they are exercising their own ultimate POWER over themselves to do so.

Still, external resources teach us to believe the contradiction to factual reality directing us, instead, our duty as concerned PERSONS is to attempt to extract other people's RESPONSIBILITY (accountability) for themselves, attach it to us and take care of it as though it were our own. They tell us to be properly caring PERSONS, we are expected, obediently, to accomplish this impossible goal. Conforming as instructed, much like mechanical robots, even when we are not externally performing tasks to take care of others, we continue to practice our taught duty internally by feeling punitively guilty.

The gut-level agreement to accept the unrealistic assignment is apparent when we hear ourselves thinking and verbalizing such statements as:

> "If it weren't for me ….";
> "If only I had …":
> "What if I had done/said/felt ….";
> "I ought to feel ashamed because I did/said/felt ____"; etc

The punitive guilt feelings above have been defined by external teachers with such untrue meanings as:

- we are at fault or to blame for choices others make for their thoughts, feelings and behaviors (crazy-producing attempts to possess power over the attitude of others); and
- we should, have to, ought to, etc. (crazy extreme words) feel uncomfortable—preferably punitively guilty—about consequences the other encounters resulting from their choices (crazy-producing pressuring extreme words).

Unhealthily, we learn to perceive ourselves as having committed near criminal offenses when, despite obedient and diligent endeavors, our other-responsibility role repeatedly is not successful. Regardless of this truth, we proceed to tell ourselves such statements as:

> "_____ (she/he) that I have been so concerned about has just done _____ to injure/embarrass/ disrespect, etc. themselves and it's all my fault! Where did all of my teaching and influence (e.g., power) go?"

Well, frankly speaking, how ridiculously inaccurate to believe and feel we ever had such power over someone else!

In contrast to learned expectations, real-life instances consistently demonstrate others continue to:

- think and make decisions for themselves (e.g., retain their POWER of AUTHORITY); and
- regulate the thoughts, feelings and behaviors they select (e.g., maintain their POWER of CONTROL).

Since the three components of genuine POWER are inseparable, how then ... realistically ... can we pluck ... selectively and exclusively... another person's inherent

POWER of RESPONSIBILITY from them without also extracting the other two POWER components?!?

Regardless of external teachings, definitions and our most sincere efforts, people intuitively know on our feelings-level of wisdom we are not capable of possessing genuine RESPONSIBILITY for someone/thing external to ourselves. Besides, even if remotely such a transplant could occur, it would be dead weight to carry without also acquiring ownership of its two indivisible traveling companions.

We can be:

> interested in;
> caring/concerned about;
> influential with (only with their permission);
> considerate of;
> thoughtful about; etc.

However, each of us ultimately flips our own internal switches to make final choices for happenings occurring in our thoughts, feelings and behaviors. In addition, the switch-flipper—SELF—experiences the greatest amount of after-effects or consequences resulting from our behavioral selections.

PERSONAL POWER is authentic, but limited in effective range to SELF exclusively. Devoting time and energy toward expanding this reality will forever remain useless endeavors—regardless of our most diligent efforts and/or another person's sincere delegations of blame.

Crazy-Producing Theme # 2: Sacrifice SELF—Always

In decoding its supportive transmissions, it was apparent from workshop contributors that constructive guilt carries another healthy message for our attention. After describing how we get ourselves into emotional imbalance—by working futilely to acquire ownership of genuine RESPONSIBILITY for others—its arousal also confirms for us when:

- we are successful in our effort to be RESPONSIBLE for ourselves—first by "placing SELF—first" on this occasion.

Restated, in addition to validating we are not endeavoring to be responsible for inclusions in another person's attitude, another healthy message is signaled by the emotion's prominence. Its presence supportively reassures us:

when we have corrected our stress-producing behavior,

assumed RESPONSIBILITY for our own emotional health and
successfully accomplished "placing ourselves—first",
at least in this instance.

Intuitively we know on our emotional level some amount of SELF-first behavior is mandatory for healthy emotional development and maintenance. This is innately-known knowledge included in the CORE of our humanness. However, external resources advocate the adoption of an "others-first—always" platform. The key thought here is "always".

With due respect, the concept of "others—first" has some merit. When we live among other people, practicing "SELF—first" behaviors the majority of the time is equally as unhealthy emotionally as spending the bulk of our time engaging in "others—first" behaviors. Common sense dictates any attitudinal activity practiced to an extreme is harmful and results in illness.

However,

- to eliminate our option to exercise PERSONAL CHOICE in matters (e.g., sometimes "SELF—first", other times "others—first") and

- in attempts to achieve complete control over us (partial control, outsiders are aware, is ineffective),

external teachers demandingly add emphasis and pressure to the "others—first" rule for living. They attach a how-to from their team of extreme words designed to restrict or erase PERSONAL CHOICE: "always". Subsequently, the rule we are urged to adopt mandates:

"others first—always",

moving it into an unbalanced, crazy-producing dimension, carrying emotionally uncomfortable outcomes for us to experience as our rewards for compliance.

Simple deduction illuminates by consenting to "place/please others first—always", the only remaining positions for ourselves are second-to-last: "SELF later—always". In effect, we are simultaneously agreeing to sacrifice ourselves—always, e.g., our own wants and preferences, and devote time and energy satisfying the wants and whims of others (people, institutions, things, etc.). Our own desires are left stranded, alone and hurting from personal neglect until some vague future time—if they are ever addressed at all!

What a gigantic "Ouch!" to our SELF-esteem and personal well-BEING.

In our society, those who elect on occasions to permit ourselves first place positions get labels assigned carrying derogatory connotations to describe us, such as:

> selfish
> inconsiderate
> not nice;
> conceited; etc.

Conversely, those who steadfastly practice the "others first—always" rule are externally applauded as:

> big; understanding
> nice/sweet;
> all giving/all-loving/all-caring;
> "all" for others, "nothing" for SELF.

Regardless of the increasing internal pressure we experience from growing collections of stressful feelings (e.g., resentment, fatigue, anger, hurt, etc) while working to achieve the crazy goal, we continue to perform the behaviors, unhealthily:

> whatever others request
> at any time the requests are issued or observed,
> we must … always … attend to (translation: feel responsible for)

their issues—first and
simultaneously,
"sacrifice ourselves—always".

For confirming information (FYI), watch the reactions of outsiders when you refuse, at times, to adhere to these externally-sanctioned guides. Your actions are judged by society as crimes, punishable preferably by huge quantities of punitive guilt.

Realistically, there is nothing wrong, criminal, sinful, etc. about practicing "SELF—first" behaviors. By doing so, the resulting guilt feelings are supportively telecasting to us the message, our proof, we have accomplished our health-producing "SELF—first" objective on that occasion. Therefore, we can <u>appreciate</u> the emotion's appearance.

Still, regardless of the FACTS, each of us retains the prerogative—the CHOICE—to continue to judge "SELF—first" behaviors as unacceptable and proceed to punish ourselves for purported crimes as we have been taught. Be aware, however, in doing so we are encouraging our guilt feeling to grow from a supportive dimension to punitive. Delivering helpful information constitutes a major part of the emotion's job description and it will defiantly grow—into a negative, unhealthy proportion if warranted—in attempts to yell its supportive messages to us even louder!

According to external teachers, as outcomes of our SELF-sacrifice practices, we are supposed to (crazy extreme word) feel good and worthwhile as a PERSON. Factually, seldom do such results occur. While we may receive external endorsements for "others first—always" behaviors, physically we are exhausted, emotionally spent and hurting from personal neglect.

One persuasion tactic utilized by external resources to influence adoption of the crazy "others first—always" platform is to generalize their opinion to the masses. We are taught everyone practices other-responsibility and SELF-sacrifice behaviors "all" of the time. The implication is while we are busily taking-on responsibility for someone/thing else, the same or another outsider is graciously on stand-by anxiously available … always … to sacrifice their wants thereby enabling them to receive our donations of responsibility for us.

Again, inherently we are aware we require some amount of SELF-first behavior for healthy emotional maintenance. While external resources promote "others first—always" as the best way to achieve emotional comfort—and we elect to try-it-on-for-size—innately we know our practices are not netting us the pleasant feelings-outcomes as predicted. Though we "try harder" (crazy extreme word) to comply with the external mandate, our personal wants are consistently left unattended. The quota of positive attention we require is not being addressed by anyone— not even ourselves.

On our feelings level, we notice, particularly during our exhaustion, our promised rescuer—the outsider to whom we have delegated the job of being responsible for our feel-good, is nowhere around. At this point, our guilt changes into resentment. In explosions of retaliation, we practice:

1) getting irritable, cranky and snappy with anyone making that "last straw" request of us;
2) vehemently blaming others for our uncomfortable feelings (e.g., "If it weren't for you …!)
3) secretly collecting emotional blackmail stamps to use for manipulating the other person(s) into feeling punitively guilty;
4) abruptly terminating relationships after accumulating strikes against the other person(s); etc.

Guilt's messages often appear confusing in that it can be the beginning of a cycle of unpleasant emotions. Regularly, it is accompanied by resentment, anger and hurt. When exploring one emotion during personal counseling sessions, another would emerge or "pop out" to relay its FACTS, only to be "up-staged" or overshadowed by yet another emotion.

The cycle of uncomfortable feelings accompanying guilt has been insightfully explained by ordinary people as follows:

1. We admit to attempting to practice our socially-assigned duty to be responsible for others first—always (guilt).

7. only to be replaced by guilt, again, for feeling resentful of our obligation to always help "helpless" others first!

2. Momentarily, we resent our obligation to take care of them, while forced to neglect ourselves.

6. Resentment for the imposition of having to get angry rapidly follows,

3. Resentment is a form of anger, that, in turn,

5. Soon, we become angry because we are hurting.

▶4. signals the presence of personal hurt.   ▲

Without effective intervention, the cycle is repeated and our collection of hurts ... from SELF-omissions ... increases

… with each repetition … towards their next explosive outburst.

Look again at the cycle of unpleasant emotions. Observe the flood of crazy extreme words permeating throughout:

> duty (expected to);
> obligation (should);
> forced (have to);
> obligation (ought to, supposed to);
> always (never refuse);
> having to (must).

Extreme words strive diligently to eliminate PERSONAL CHOICE. Their exclusive job is to encourage us to forget our permanently available options to "place SELF—first" at times and "others—first" at other times.

Let's move on to another related issue pertaining to guilt

Believing the myth AUTHORITY, RESPONSIBILITY or CONTROL can be exchanged among people establishes the basic foundation for emotional manipulation, also known as emotional blackmail.

EMOTIONAL BLACKMAIL

Emotional blackmail is usually a one-sided emotional game wherein another person believes, on their feelings-level, they have extorted a segment of our innate POWER over our thoughts, feelings and behaviors. Impossibly, they attach it onto themselves. In exchange, they assign their POWER segment(s) to us. To illustrate, using the example of exchanges of POWER of RESPONSIBILITY:

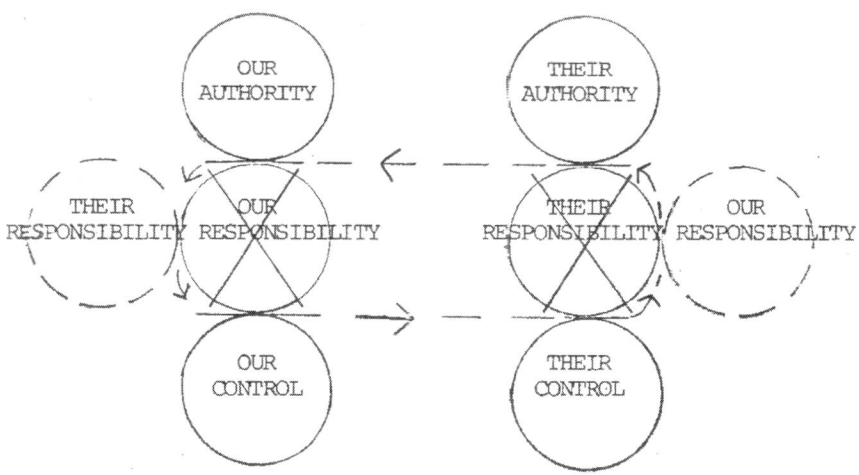

POWER OVER OURSELVES and ANOTHER'S POWER OVER THEMSELVES

Whether or not we are aware of the game-playing scheme, the game proceeds as follows:

- The annexed segment of power over us grants them the privilege, they believe, to manipulate any and all

POWER segments over our attitude whenever they choose to do so.

- Conjointly, they donate their POWER components to us entitling them to credit/blame us for all happenings occurring in their attitude.
- Subsequent to the exchange of POWERS, whatever they:

> entertain as thoughts,
> experience as feelings and/or
> perform as behaviors

are attributed to us. In addition, keep in mind, along with their exchange-of- POWER strategy, the extortionist harbors the unrealistic belief they own our genuine POWER and have the ability to maneuver our thoughts, feelings and behaviors.

Though their emotional blackmail scheme is crazy, as long as we agree to react/perform as they desire, the atmosphere between the two of us is pleasant. When we feel good, they take the credit; when they feel good, we get the credit. However, when they feel bad, we are at fault or to blame, and they implement a plan to force us to feel punitively guilty or accountable for their pain. Feeling punitively guilty is the ransom they believe we must pay for the crime we have committed against them. Payment is demanded using such statements as:

"After all I've done for you!"
"See what you made me do/feel/think!"
"I can't believe you did/said that in front of me!"
"How could you do this to me?!?"

When we cooperate and respond to their "feel guilty" mandates by feeling punitively guilty and complying with their demands for our behavior, they take credit for their power over us and feel better—temporarily.

Truthfully speaking, emotional blackmail schemes become ineffective the moment we decide against allowing ourselves to be unhealthily manipulated. In addition, the anger and resentment the blackmailing person often experience following our refusal to feel guilty as they command are signaling realistic, helpful messages to their attention and ours:

1) the power they believed they owned over us does not exist; and
2) they are hurting themselves by clinging to the crazy belief they can actually acquire ownership of any segment of our innate POWER over ourselves!

Personal Pain Signaled by GUILT

Although we may be slow to admit it, a portion of the resentment and anger accompanying guilt results from our neglect of SELF. Consistently ranking our wants as "last" or ignoring our preferences entirely, becomes painful after a while, rather than pleasant as externally-predicted. While devoting our time and attention to "pleasing others first—always", the job of taking care of ourselves reads "Vacancy".

Repeatedly responding with "No!" to our own requests for SELF-first attentions simultaneously stimulates emotional hurt for us to endure. Although we have learned to believe differently, the feelings-level of our humanness remains aware, intuitively, some amount of SELF-first behavior is required from us for our own healthy, comfortable emotional maintenance. Without the quota needed from ourselves, our emotional status is precariously at risk.

In the interest of balance, there are instances when, after honest evaluations, we may agree our SELF-first actions were inconsiderate of others. Still, it is important to determine the amount of punitive guilt to experience so that it corresponds to the offense we have committed. In fairness to ourselves, we need to adjust the intensity of guilt and length of time we emotionally suffer, according to a reasonable assessment of the facts presented by both people involved—ourselves and the other person(s).

In addition, look at each situation as an independent instance, rather than combining it with others from our past.

PUNISHMENT WITH PUNITIVE GUILT FEELINGS = WEIGHT OF OFFENSE!

This system of metering justice functions well in the everyday legal world and it can also reestablish balance in our daily emotional world.

If you are one who has allowed yourself to be controlled by punitive guilt, you can break the habit. Get started by deliberately practicing giving yourself a genuine CHOICE in situations as they occur. Remember, the social systems neither support nor condemn personal sanity, comfort and emotionally balanced living. They merely state their positions and opinions. Opinions are not the same as FACTS. Opinions are subject to errors and mistakes in judgment, while FACTS persist eternally truthful and unchanged.

To break the habit of permitting others to manipulate you with guilt, as you experience the emotion, ask yourself and honestly answer:

"What is the crime I have committed? Does it warrant punishment?"

After answering the question:

1. If you decide feeling punitively guilty is appropriate for you,
   a.) Set a time limit to experience the feeling. As example, say to yourself, "I agree to feel guilty for one hour (day, week, etc.)"
   b.) Then set the clock, literally if necessary, to alarm at the end on one hour (or mark the calendar to display whatever span of time you allocate for feeling guilty).
   c.) During that time-span, concentrate your energy on feeling punitively guilty.
   d.) When the time expires, force yourself to get involved in a pre-determined fun activity you sincerely enjoy to redirect your energy towards feeling better.

2. If you determine you have sacrificed a personal want for yourself, give yourself another want to substitute. Examples of alternates:
   - play a favorite DVD and shadow-dance with yourself;

- soak in a bubble bath with candles surrounding;
- wash your hair if that feels good;
- phone a supportive friend;
- buy yourself a plant or a long-wanted toy;
- cook your favorite meal, or go out to a favorite restaurant;
- play a round of golf; basketball at the gym; go for a drive in the country;
- take yourself to a movie;
- write yourself a love letter and read it aloud while standing before a mirror;
- go swimming; relax beside a body of water; etc.

3. If you choose not to honor another person's request to put them first at this particular time:
    - inform them without feeling obligated to supply them with explanations. Saying, "I'd rather not" is sufficient.
    - Then, when you feel guilt's presence, reinterpret its meaning as a positive signal you have actually placed yourself first—and that is emotionally healthy!

Remember, the other person is capable of finding another solution to their problem, just as they decided to use you as their answer.

4. If you decide to honor another's request first:
    Let yourself know what you are doing with full awareness. You are choosing to sacrifice your want on this occasion in their favor. By respecting our own right to have a CHOICE in the matter, we reduce the amount of resentment and anger scheduled to flow later.

Relinquishing guilt as a constant companion represents a change from our usual pattern of everyday living. Change means death of the familiar and birth of the unfamiliar. When it occurs, there is a loss and as such, we will grieve for the familiar—regardless of the unhealthy and painful consequences we have suffered.

In preparation for making changes in your usual feelings, we respectfully suggest you review the discussions from earlier during this tour on "Change and the Change Process" and "Grieving"—its naturally-flowing aftermath.

<u>WORRY</u>

Worry emanates from fear. As a card-carrying permanent member of our inherently complete set of feelings, it, too, signals useful and beneficial information to support a healthy emotional status for its owner.

Worry is our innate clue alerting us the problem-solving process we are using to reduce our fear is incomplete. As previously reported on this tour, fear signals three basic messages, namely, we:

> lack trustworthy information;
> lack preparation; and
> lack protection.

The encouraging message from worry is telling us, while we have assembled some amount of trustworthy information—through identifying negative events that can possibly happen related to an issue—we have yet to prepare ourselves just in case those outcomes occur. Consequently, signals worry, we have left ourselves without preparation and protection from identified unpleasant outcomes. Finishing the process involves preparing or completing a realistic action-plan to address as many potential problem-issues as we can recognize in advance.

Therefore, in healthy amounts, the emotion is informing us about a deficiency existing in the resolution phase towards diminishing our fear.

To complete the fear-resolution process, our plan of action needs to delineate:

- specific things we can actually Do to prevent, where possible, the undesirable events from occurring;
- remedial actions we can realistically implement in the event the negatives transpire; and/or
- acceptance of our limitations and inability to Do anything to prevent or remedy some of the problem-outcomes considered.

Characteristically, worry is future-related and negative-oriented. Our attention is frozen on the question "What if _____ happens?" and we fill-in the blank with a series of negatives or undesirable prospective outcomes. Absent from the process is follow-through to plan "then I will Do _____ to prepare myself for my protection".

Generally, we have little difficulty deciphering possible negative outcomes that can take place related to any activity or endeavor. Unpleasant aftermaths occupy a significant portion of our knowledge-base. The accumulation of "Be Scared" messages is gathered from personal experiences and external teaching resources throughout living. Still, for balance, remember on the other side of the coin resides positive conceivable end results also eternally present and available for experiencing. We can reach them faster by planning how-to's to overcome the identified negatives in advance, thereby clearing and paving the pathway to secure the positives.

In healthy amounts, worry functions as a motivator for productive thinking and protective planning. By

- listening to worry's advance warnings; and
- sorting or flowing with the emotion to determine workable solutions or how-to's for our actions, if needed,

we can significantly reduce the amount of scare and anxiety we live with daily.

While it is true we can neither predict the future nor achieve total control over it, we do have the ability to hinder many of the experiences we could possibly later encounter and significantly influence (not the same as "control") the method of presentation of several others. You are aware the actions we practice today yield results we experience tomorrow and into our future.

Practicing behaviors today that point to personal support and protection

bring their rewards
later in time
for us to enjoy.
    Deciding to refrain from or discontinue practices

that weigh heavily toward trouble-territory for us
later,
also includes a decision to avoid
many of the negative consequences
accompanying those behaviors.

In addition, being aware of our current behavior
(including emotional behavior)
as unhealthy or non-profitable for us
and electing to Do nothing to correct it,
also means deciding to experience repeatedly
the corresponding unpleasant results
continuously lurking around
to endure in the future.

In flowing positively with the emotion, many personal development participants agree worry signals its message to us with supportive instructions summarized into three parts:

Part 1: collect/assemble information;

Part 2: prepare ourselves; and

Part 3: provide protection for ourselves.

The popular, though unhealthy practice of lingering on Part-one of worry's instructions, without following-through to Parts two and three, constitutes an incomplete message-transmission. Therefore, despite the volume of information we foresee with our "What if (negative outcome) happens?" projections, the feeling of worrying will not effectively shrink or disappear.

From an earlier discussion, you can recall:

- once an emotion has gleaned information from our external and internal worlds and
- becomes "on alert" or aroused inside us;
- it is bound by duty—assigned by our Creator—
- to complete the second part of its purpose for arousal:
 … the message-delivering function.

Our uncomfortable emotion cannot feel better until it knows, intuitively, it has achieved delivering the message it carries for our consideration. Consequently, rather than subsiding in defeat to its at rest position inside us, our feeling of worry will insultingly swell—often to excessive and unhealthy proportions.

Chronic worriers have a highly developed pace for outlining unpleasant potential end-results. Unfortunately, large segments of valuable time are spent fearfully fixated at "Part-one" of worry's healthy instructions. Rather than moving-on to formulating protective solutions for themselves, their energy is devoted to refining and providing more details to identified problems.

With sufficient practice or repetition in identifying negative outcomes that can possibly happen—without following-through to SELF-protective solutions—unhealthily we improve our ability to worry. In addition, the absence of solutions to anticipated problems is fertile soil for the innate seeds of scare and anxiety to grow. As a result, we endure an overdose of fear and anxiety about most issues.

Regarding a related issue involving the feeling of worry, during workshops several people shared they learned to perceive worrying as a demonstration of affection for another person/thing. For them, the emotion has been incorrectly redefined as symbolic "proof of caring". The unhealthy guideline for living misinforms by advising when we genuinely care about someone or something, we are supposed to (crazy extreme word) worry about them. The more we care, the greater our worrying practices ought to (crazy extreme word) become.

Along with this belief comes the additional myth suggesting, to demonstrate affectionate feelings for another, we have to (crazy extreme word) feel uncomfortable ourselves—a theme harboring the unattractive underlying message: "love is painful"! What an inverted, incongruent twist to reality! Unfortunately, while practicing the untrue guideline—in sincere efforts to indirectly express our interest and caring for another—

> simultaneously we move ourselves
> from a point of healthy concern
> into personally-debilitating worrying.

Exploring the "worry equals caring" theory in more depth with participants, it became apparent in most instances when worrying about another, as in guilt, we are attempting to take charge of genuine RESPONSIBILITY for them— an impossible task for us to achieve. In addition, we are striving to exercise power over events the other person could potentially encounter, in useless efforts to prevent negative occurrences from happening. You can recall from an earlier discussion during this tour, RESPONSIBILITY is a segment of the authentic POWER every individual permanently retains over ourselves, but no-one and no-thing else.

The misguiding belief we are practicing implies, to prove we care, our task is to guarantee the other's safety and security. Since it is clear our physical capability to protect them is limited, prohibiting us from literally carrying out the assignment, ingeniously we decide to master the duty emotionally through worrying, mingled intermittenly with feelings of punitive guilt.

While POWER over our attitude is complete and unlimited, we absolutely cannot expand its capabilities to annex and/or manipulate either segment of another's POWER over their attitude. Regardless of the most ardent efforts, every human being eternally owns the innate abilities and ultimate privilege of managing our own POWER in whatever manner we choose. Conjointly, we also possess the unique privilege to experience consequences accompanying our chosen thoughts, feelings and behaviors—pleasant as well as unpleasant aftermaths, dependent upon our selections.

In actuality, despite the dimensions of our love for another, our ability to safeguard their future is restricted to being:

> interested in them;
> influential with them (only with their permission);
> caring for them;
> concerned about them;
> supportive of them; etc.

Continued efforts to assume responsibility for them on any level of human existence are personal set-ups for failure.

Rather than persisting with the impossible duties and worrying excessively, it would be to our emotional advantage to return our collections of assumed power to their inherent owners. Authentic RESPONSIBILITY (accountability) for outcomes of an external event another encounters is shared between that other person/thing and the situation.

As it relates to the event, there are factors contributing to outcomes brought about by the situation itself and, realistically, we cannot be accountable for them. Included among these factors are:

- the time of day an outcome occurs;
- the geographical location—or where it happens;
- existing weather conditions at the time it presents;
- the level of oxygen available;
- electrical/mechanical functions and malfunctions;
- location of surrounding objects in the outcome's setting;
- exact method of presentation the outcome manifests; etc.

Regarding the other person, we cannot be genuinely RESPONSIBLE (ACCOUNTABLE) for their:

- thoughts, feelings, mannerisms and other behaviors;
- reaction processes and methods of SELF regulation;
- biases, prejudices, likes and dislikes;
- talents, skills, shortcomings, mistakes made;
- hopes, dreams, expectations of themselves/us; etc.

For clarification, let us interject here that excessive worry is to be differentiated from having a healthy concern for our own, a situation's, or another person's well-BEING. Though worry and concern are similar in some respects, they are dramatically different in others.

True, while experiencing both emotions, we engage in:

- anticipating negative possible outcomes and perhaps
- conjuring up possible solutions the other person (or we) can employ

to avoid and/or remedy these unpleasant events.

As differences, however,

in healthy concern, we	while in excessive worry, we
express our projections and preferences for their behavior, while remaining aware our opinions are not absolutes;	express our projections and behavioral preferences for them, while expecting the other to think, feel and behave as we prefer;
encourage them to think and to assume RESPONSIBILITY for themselves, e.g., we urge them to review pros and cons of available options for their behavior;	refuse to acknowledge the other's inherent RIGHT and ability to think and develop plans for themselves (or we deny our own abilities to think and plan for ourselves);
allow the other person to make plans in the interest of their own welfare, and respect their decisions (this does not mean we "have to" agree with their choices);	discount their decisions— implying they are helpless nitwits requiring our skilled guidelines and projections (or, we discount our ability to help ourselves);
exercise RESPONSIBILITY for our own welfare by formulating specific plans to protect our own integrity—in the event we, or the other person encounter trouble;	repeatedly caution and advise them (or ourselves) to beware, and covertly, to "be scared";

let-go of our uncomfortable feeling and	cling to our unpleasant feeling and
move-on to other issues occurring in our own life.	remain afraid for them (or ourselves) throughout our daily living experiences.
In essence, we accept our limitations in ability to manage another person's life, and redirect our time and efforts to the feasible realm of managing ourselves.	In effect, we continue our useless attempts to manipulate the other's future, while ignoring our realistic POWER to healthily manage ourselves now and later.

Worrying, practiced exclusively, neither prepares nor protects us from unpleasant potential outcomes. It simply identifies them for us. Following-through to formulate plans we can realistically implement are concrete steps toward effectively managing ourselves today and in the future. Simultaneously, we reduce the intensity of our feeling of worry with each realistic action-plan developed.

Breaking the habit of worrying excessively requires deliberate efforts initially in practicing exchanging well-formed thoughts, feelings and behaviors for newly selected ones we are substituting towards a healthy change. Regardless of how difficult it may seem to implement at first trial, the new behaviors become easier and easier with repeated practice ... over time ... in using them—guaranteed!

Change means death of the familiar and birth of the unfamiliar. Whenever it occurs, we experience a loss. Despite being aware the loss is to our benefit, we will grieve the departure of our familiar.

When you decide to implement sincere steps toward changing your worrying habit, we believe it would be helpful, in preparation, to review previous discussions on "Change and the Change Process" and "Grieving"—the naturally-flowing aftermath of change.

<u>FRUSTRATION</u>

Frustration occupies a permanent residence among our inherent set of emotions. Similar to its emotional colleagues, when aroused, it signals useful information in support of our overall well-BEING.

Frustration healthily signals:

> an obstacle or block is present and interfering with our efforts to achieve a desired goal.

There is an obstruction in the pathway hindering (not the same as preventing) progress towards our identified want.

In addition, the emotion instructs us with how-to's for its resolution:

- review the steps in our action-plan;
- modify them as needed or formulate different ones;
- implement the changes;
- evaluate our progress within a reasonable time-frame.

Everyone encounters obstacles occasionally throughout daily living. Sometimes we can anticipate the blocks and even predict them, while at other times they appear unannounced and quite unexpected. Whenever they manifest themselves, they are disturbing and upsetting.

Obstructions, in themselves, cannot prevent us from accomplishing a goal. We may, however, be required to develop an alternate route or action- plan-#2 involving additional and/or different steps towards its attainment. Still, as a cardinal rule:

—as long as the goal is realistic and attainable—

it remains eternally available to us, ready and willing to be claimed.

When reviewed objectively and positively, frustration presents opportunity for personal growth. To enhance continuous upward progression, it can motivate us to:

- determine who/what is blocking our path;
- assess what they are saying and doing (or not doing) to influence us to feel blocked;
- broaden our knowledge through researching for additional/alternate resources available;
- review and evaluate positive aspects and rewards associated with the goal;
- make decisions on workable how-to's to remove the block or circumvent it;
- implement corrective plans;
- take credit for steps taken en route;
- evaluate our progress throughout the process and upon goal achievement.

In addition to using our positive qualities and realistic abilities, among outside resources to possibly assist are:

- other people with specific expertise and skills used as consultants and mentors, along with their involvement to an extent;

- financial resources and institutions for funding;
- books and other printed literature;
- internet and other electronic media; etc.

Keep in mind, for our want to be achievable, it needs to be within our realm of genuine POWER to accomplish. In the real world, authentic POWER over attitudes (thoughts, feelings and behaviors) is limited to SELF alone. We literally cannot expand our capabilities to govern and manage the attitude of another person/thing external to ourselves.

Let's take a look at the negative benefits and uses of frustration.

Often people learn to manipulate others and their environment by appearing helpless when they experience frustration. To them, depending upon others for assistance is easier and faster towards achieving a goal than relying upon SELF. They sacrifice their own intelligence among other strengths, creating an unhealthy dependency upon others for their welfare. Independent functioning is side-stepped and looked upon as a burden destined to flop/fail.

Such lack of SELF-confidence is fertile ground for constructive frustration to grow to unhealthy, destructive and stressful proportions.

As long as they elect to continue to portray helplessness, they simultaneously disown their own uniqueness and special talents, while denying themselves direct personal fulfillments. They cheat themselves from experiencing the inner glows, warmth and thrilling sensations stemming from personal goal-achievement. "I did it, myself!" feels a great deal better emotionally than "You did it for me".

Realistically, there does not exist a legitimate reason for remaining frustrated. The emotion is merely a signal—not a cause. Its' etiology is lack of knowledge and implementing non-productive steps yielding limited progress for you.

If this scenario describes you, allow yourself the opportunity to get out of the dependency trap. Remember, you already own every trait and ability required to achieve any realistic goal you desire. The qualities remain eternally available for your use simply because you are human, whenever you alertly decide to use them.

To repeat for emphasis, there is no quality or ability missing from your humanness preventing you from taking charge of your own life and the consequences of your choices. True, you may not have deliberately used them until this point, but they remain a part of you and accessible. You may feel as though in quantity or amount the qualities are the size of a mustard seed. However, that amount of the quality is 100% yours—forever. With practice in its use, it can expand to a larger dimension.

If this scenario describes someone you know to whom you have served, unhealthily, as their enabler, there is a more beneficial pathway for you to employ. Begin relinquishing your role by refraining from answering every question asked by the dependent person. Instead, encourage their resourcefulness. Direct them to other resources to find answers (e.g., books, internet, experts in that area, bankers, magazines, etc.). Ask for a report of their findings within a reasonable time-limit to receive the report. Then compliment their efforts when their report—partial or complete—is received.

To avoid frustration's dependency trap or to get out of it, here are some suggestions for consideration when feelings of frustration arrive. Before asking others for help, take some time to ask and honestly answer for yourself such questions as:

1. Who or what does the block consist of?
    You are specifically identifying the block.
2. What is the block's message to you:
    What is the block saying to you and doing (or not doing) to influence you to feel hindered.

Provide an answer to each message contained in the block. Example: Block says "So you want to be an artist. You can't draw a straight line!"

You answer "But I can make beautiful linking curves. When I need a straight line, I'll get a ruler!"

3. Make decisions on workable how-to's for resolving the conflict where possible.

   What are some things you can actually Do now and later to get past this obstruction? Begin with small steps you can take and progress to larger ones.

4. Implement your corrective plans.

5. Evaluate your progress at pre-set intervals remembering to take credit for steps completed.

6. Enjoy the end-results and again take credit at the goal's completion.

This is your life and your future. No one else can live it better than you. You know your wants, preferences and your comfortable pace for implementing steps toward your goals. So, get started achieving what you really want from your own endeavors.

As you implement sincere steps to relieve frustration, you can anticipate some amount of grief from death of the block. Though its departure is a desired one, it constitutes a loss. As such, you will likely mourn its leaving.

It would be beneficial to review the previous discussions along this tour on "Change and the Change Process" and "Grieving" to recognize and evaluate your status towards shrinking your aroused emotion.

CONFUSION

Confusion is another valuable member of the team of emotions composing our inherent and complete set. When aroused from its resting status, the message it signals is useful information in support of our overall health.

Confusion informs us in the process of determining how to conduct ourselves in our attitude, e.g.,

> what to think,
> how to feel and
> how to behave,
>> we are listening to two or more viewpoints
>> concerning the same issue
>> for our behavior,
>> that are conflicting or clashing,
>> one with the other.

The opposing opinions are coming from one external teaching resource or several with whom we confer and trust to tell us which behavior(s) to select for practice to be a proper PERSON.

You are aware from birth throughout our lifetime, we are exposed to a barrage of instructions on how to conduct ourselves in our attitude. Teachers prevalent among our daily living environment remain constantly and loyally on stand-by, eagerly waiting to contribute their opinions to us at every opportunity. The variable points of view they readily share are presented as though they were unyielding facts, incapable of being in error—even slightly.

At times we may wish to establish credibility for some of the positions they promote. When we collect the courage to point out inconsistencies and to question the basis for the guarantees they issue, attempting to substantiate their opinions, it is not unusual for them to haughtily retort to us in anger, "How dare you question me!"

Frankly, just so you will know, their anger is a defense maneuver designed to protect them from answering us, while encouraging us to feel afraid and guilty for doubting them in the first place! Consequently, we are left as we started—with our feeling of confusion.

Perhaps at younger ages questioning inconsistencies in externally-defined directives for our behaviors was not safe for us to practice. Still, we can take full credit for the SELF-protective measures used then and thank ourselves for selecting them. Whether healthy or unhealthy, at least the measures assisted us in surviving emotionally until now.

To heighten your awareness, let's try-on an interviewing exercise demonstrating the conflicting advise and instructions relayed by external resources on how to manage our attitude. We will screen a behavioral question through several environmental teachers and listen to their answers (e.g., our taught guidelines) silently or state them aloud.

BEHAVIOR QUESTION	EXTERNAL TEACHING RESOURCES	TAUGHT GUIDELINES FOR OUR BEHAVIOR
	family members	Men must be brave, strong. = No
	church, religion	Medical science says its relieves pressure. = Yes
Can a man cry and still be masculine?	schools	Of course! = Yes
	media: TV, movies	Real men never cry. = No
	songs	Only women and babies cry. = No
		Big boys don't. = No
	books, newspapers, magazines	Shows you care. = Yes
		According to Readers Digest…. = Maybe

252

jobs and personnel manuals, policies co-workers	You look so ugly when you cry. = No Enter into thy closet = Maybe
neighbors government, public laws, ethical codes etiquette	Jesus wept. = Yes Try harder not to = No No! Means you are out of control. = No
specialists, experts	Makes others uncomfortable = Maybe At funerals only = Maybe Feels better than keeping hurts inside. = Yes

Look again at the column of guidelines. Is it apparent a conflict exists among the advocated solutions? A summary of the responses by external teachers is a definite "maybe" as the answer to the question and maybe's are unclear, baffling, noncommittal and confusing!

You might be wondering by this point: Is there a way to resolve this dilemma and arrive at a comfortable decision to practice—at least for now? Personal development workshop participants have repeatedly shared an emphatic "Yes!" There is a way that works to our emotional benefit. From the gamut of possible options for our behavior ... and their inseparable teammates—their consequences ... each person can determine for ourselves which solutions feel the most comfortable for us to practice during a given situation and place.

Regardless of the discomfort we may experience in doing so, the unique ability to reduce our confusion belongs to ourselves—exclusively. We retain the prerogative and realistic POWER to exercise this inherent privilege with awareness for ourselves whenever we CHOOSE.

Often deceptive scare and punitive guilt caution us to believe if we take steps to decrease our confusion, those who shared their opinions with us will be crushed emotionally and suffer from our actions. However, realistically, CHOOSING to shrink the confusion does not injure the teachers. You are simply removing and trashing the power they enjoyed over you. To maintain their survival, they will continue to exist another day to influence someone else into accepting their directives.

Keep in mind external teachers neither support nor condemn our sanity. They merely issue directives, based upon their opinions at the time, whether those options are consistent or not with their viewpoints shared previously.

To shrink confusion, review your thoughts and the diversity of opinions regarding a particular issue. We can evaluate the validity and usefulness of external guidelines to us today by screening them through our innate abilities:

> to think for ourselves;
> to use our intelligence and common sense;
> to weigh pros and cons before taking actions;
> to exercise good judgment now and later as warranted;
> to make new decisions in our own best interest;
> to realistically plan;
> to follow-through with our plans;
> to evaluate the results we enjoy; etc.

Summarize the present-day value of external directives and opinions by deliberately asking and answering for yourself:

> If I agree to think (feel or behave) in this manner, what is in this for me (pleasant and unpleasant outcomes)?

Let your imagination flow. The answers you summon may well provide the stimulus required to make decisions for yourself regarding your own attitudinal practices. Opinions delivered by external resources can be effectively reduced to suggestions, rather than forces allowed to control and confuse us.

When we permit ourselves the opportunity, each of us is capable of selecting behaviors to practice in our overall best interest and to our advantage. The process begins by making an alert, sincere and committed CHOICE to do so.

Again, before implementing changes in your emotional status, we believe it would be beneficial to review the discussions on "Change and the Change Process" and "Grieving", its naturally flowing aftermath. The renewed awareness will likely be helpful throughout your changes.

EPILOGUE

A STATEMENT

Emotions or feelings are integral parts of our wholeness designed by our Creator to add quality and clarity to our life. Their purposes for existing—their intrinsically-assigned jobs—are to collect valid information and deliver realistic insights to their owner concerning the internal and external worlds we live in.

Since their very survival depends upon it, emotions literally cannot rest until both parts of their duty are completed. You may be aware emotions gather information. However, successfully delivering collected information requires our cooperation in receiving and evaluating its healthy contributions toward our overall well-BEING. The more we ignore our feelings, through silence and non-involvement, we condone their growth into stressful proportions. Additionally, when we choose to refrain from exercising our genuine POWER over them to control them, we simultaneously grant permission to the emotions to collect our lucrative power donations and seemingly assume control and management over us.

While we do not have complete control over our physical body parts, emotions do not fall into the same "impossible to regulate" category. Despite appearances, each of us inherently possesses the components of genuine POWER over our attitude (thoughts, feelings and behaviors) plus PERSONAL CHOICE to manage the emotions in our complete set. In fact, our POWER never leaves us.

Emotional stress is a conquerable human disorder. We firmly believe with the new and re-kindled information, along with how-to's advanced on this tour, when practiced, will be helpful in healing and remedially assisting towards successfully controlling your emotions, just as they demonstrated their effectiveness with an assortment of ordinary people who shared their profitable experiences with us.

Our sincere hope is this brief journey through our emotional world will stimulate awareness and appreciation for emotions in their own right. Feelings really are our friends. With direct, positive and respectful attention from their owner, they can assuredly lead us along pathways to reduced emotional stress and internal peace.

Accomplishing the task, of course, is a cooperative agreement that begins with:

When Feelings Speak, LISTEN!

BIBLIOGRAPHY (ALPHABETICAL ORDER)
READING REFERENCES ONLY

Bach, Richard, Illusions: The Adventures of A Reluctant Messiah, Dell Publishing/Random House Publications, New York, New York, Copyright © 1977. All rights reserved.

Dyer, Wayne, MD, Your Erroneous Zones, Harper Collins Publishers, New York, New York 10022, Copyright © 1976. All rights reserved.

Harris, Thomas A. MD, "I'm OK—You're OK", Harper Collins Publishers, New York, New York 10022, Copyright ©1967. All rights reserved.

Hutschnecker, Arnold, MD, The Will To Live, Prentice-Hall Publishers, Upper Saddle River, New Jersey, Copyright © 1966. All rights reserved.

James, Muriel, PhD and Jongeward, Dorothy, PhD. Born To Win, Addison Wesley Publishing Company, Boston, Massachusetts 02116, Copyright © 1976. All rights reserved.

Kubler-Ross, Elizabeth, MD, <u>On Death and Dying,</u> The Macmillan Company, Hampshire RG21 6YS England, Copyright © 1969. All rights reserved.

Lair, Jess, PhD., <u>"I Ain't Much Baby, But I'm All I've Got",</u> Fawcett Publications/Random House Publications, New York, New York, Copyright © 1969. All rights reserved.

Maslow, Abraham, JD, <u>Motivation and Personality,2nd Edition,</u> Harper Collins Publishers, New York, New York 10022, Copyright © 1970. All rights reserved.

Newman, Mildred, MD and Berkowitz, Bernard, MD, <u>How To Be Your Own Best Friend,</u> Ballantine Books, Inc., New York, New York 10019, Copyright ©1971. All rights reserved.

Olson, Dr. Ken, <u>Can You Wait Till Friday?: The Psychology of Hope,</u> Fawcett Publications/Random House Publications, New York, New York, Copyright © 1975. All rights reserved.

Perls, Frederick S., MD, PhD., <u>Gestalt Therapy Verbatim,</u> Real People Press, Boulder, Colorado 80302, Copyright © 1969. All Rights reserved.

Perls, Fritz, MD, PhD., <u>The Gestalt Approach and Eye Witness to Therapy,</u> Science and Behavior Books, Palo Alto, California 94306, Copyright © 1973. All rights reserved.

Prather, Hugh, <u>Notes To Myself,</u> Real People Press, Boulder, Colorado 80302, Copyright © 1970. All rights reserved.

Rogers. Carl, PhD., <u>On Becoming A Person,</u> Houghton Mifflin Hartcourt Publishing Company, New York, New York 10003, Copyright © 1961. All rights reserved.

Selye, Hans, MD, <u>The Stress of Life,</u> McGraw-Hill Companies, New York, New York 10121, Copyright © 1956. All rights reserved.

Smith, Manuel J., PhD., <u>When I Say No, I Feel Guilty</u>, Random House Publishers, New York, New York 10019, Copyright © 1975. All rights reserved.

Steiner, Claude, PhD., <u>Scripts People Live,</u> Grove Press, Inc., New York, New York 10003, Copyright © 1974. All rights reserved.

ABOUT THE AUTHOR

Freeda L. Biggs Moore is a native of Tyler, Texas where she graduated valedictorian of her Emmett Scott High School Class. Her medical interests flowed from obtaining a Registered Nurse degree from Homer G. Phillips Diploma School of Nursing to earning a Bachelor of Science in Nursing degree, cum laude, from St. Louis University. Both institutions are in St. Louis, Missouri. After teaching Medical-Surgical Nursing in Missouri for three years, she returned to Texas and completed a Master's Degree in Psychiatric-Mental Health Nursing at Texas Woman's University, Houston Campus, Houston, Texas.

As an accomplished Advanced Practice Nurse (APN), Freeda practiced in the mental health field over thirty-five years. She helped to pioneer nursing entrepreneurship in Houston, Texas. With professional acuity and her easy-flowing personality, she became quite popular in her counseling and personal development enterprise. In addition to writing articles for newspapers, her expert comments were frequently published by other columnists.

During her career, she presented numerous mental health topics to a variety of lay, scholastic (secondary schools through graduate collegiate levels) and professional groups throughout Houston, the State of Texas and the nation. Much of the content of recordings for presentations along this tour stems from insights and responses shared by participants among these groups.

Freeda's hobbies include fishing, hunting, traveling and cooking with her husband, along with reading, and writing, among others. For over twenty-three years, she has been married to Dr. Yondell E. Moore, Sr, MD, a Dallas, Texas Urologist, presently retired.